# 72
# REASONS
# TO BE
# VEGAN

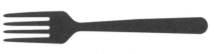

# 72

# REASONS

# TO BE

# VEGAN

## Why Plant-Based.
## Why Now.

## GENE STONE &
## KATHY FRESTON

Workman Publishing ▪▪▪ New York

Library of Congress Cataloging-in-Publication Data is available.

ISBN 978-1-5235-1031-3

Design by Rae Ann Spitzenberger
Front cover illustration: **Shutterstock:** koblizeek.
Back cover illustrations: (from left to right)
**Adobe Stock:** Togrul Babayev, pandavector, martialred.
Back flap illustration: **Adobe Stock:** Рудой Максим.
Interior illustrations: **Adobe Stock:** Arcady, p. 75; Togrul Babayev, p. 153; bitontawan02, p. 90; Comauthor, pp. 156, 161; Dshnrgc, p. 48; Elena Garder, p. 61; jiaking1, p. 183; Vlad Klok, pp. 80, 108, 116; lynea, pp. 51, 61; Рудой Максим, pp. 42, 66, 174; manstock007, p. 27; martialred, pp. 65, 149; nicknik93759375, p. 103; pandavector, pp. 24, 33; Moch Solikin, p. 13; supanut, p. 93; sviatoslav, p. 103; Tartila, p. 55; viktorinka, pp. 61, 82, 108, 116; VKA, p. 128; ylivdesign, pp. 16, 138. **Shutterstock:** koblizeek, pp. iii, 189.

*DISCLAIMER: The information in this book is not meant to replace medical advice. If you have questions about your diet, contact your physician and/or your nutritionist.*

Workman books are available at special discounts when purchased in bulk for premiums and sales promotions as well as for fund-raising or educational use. Special editions or book excerpts can also be created to specification. For details, contact the Special Sales Director at specialmarkets@workman.com.

Workman Publishing Co., Inc.
225 Varick Street
New York, NY 10014-4381
workman.com

WORKMAN is a registered trademark
of Workman Publishing Co., Inc.

Printed in Thailand
First printing February 2021

10 9 8 7 6 5 4 3 2 1

# Contents

Introduction **1**

**01** Veganism Is Happening in a Very Major Way **6**

**02** Cows Burp and Fart = Methane = Climate Change **8**

**03** It's Cheaper and Better Than Buying a Tesla **9**

**04** Soy Is Protective Against Breast Cancer (and Won't Give Guys Man Boobs) **11**

**05** Cow's Milk Is Kind of Gross **17**

**06** Your Skin Will Look Amazing **19**

**07** Fiber Is Your Body's Bitch **21**

**08** Dairy Doesn't Do a Body Good **23**

**09** Antibiotic Resistance Is No Joke **26**

**10** Dude, Your Erections #BetterLonger **28**

**11** Gals, Your Clitoris #Orgasms **29**

**12** Most Fish Are Polluted by Mercury and Plastic **30**

**13** Healthy Fats Come from Nuts, Seeds, and Avocados **32**

**14** We Can Solve World Hunger **34**

**15** You Could Be the Next Gandhi, da Vinci, or Tolstoy **36**

**16** The Keto Diet Shortens Your Life **38**

**17** Iron Is Necessary. But It Takes Plants to Get It Right. **41**

**18** We Aren't Lions **44**

**19** Eggs Are Not Incredible or Edible **46**

**20** Go Fish. No Fish. **49**

**21** Farmed Fish Are Not Going to Save Wild Fish **52**

**22** Rain Forests Are the Lungs of the Planet **54**

**23** We're Running Out of Water **57**

**24** The Numbers Don't Lie **59**

**25** Animals Deserve Better **62**

**26** Meat and Dairy Addiction Is Real **64**

**27** You Can Live Long and Prosper **67**

**28** Plant Protein Is Clean Protein **69**

**29** Your Gut Will Thank You **73**

**30** Martinis. Coffee. Fun. **76**

**31** The World Is Becoming Overrun with Animal Poop **79**

**32** There Is No Such Thing as Humane Slaughter **81**

**33** Working at a Slaughterhouse Is Hell **84**

**34** Laughing Gas Is Not So Funny **87**

**35** It's Good for Growing Kids! **88**

**36** You Want to Live Longer Than a Caveman **92**

**37** You Can Up Your Game **95**

**38** Creamy Doesn't Have to Mean Dairy **98**

**39** Foodborne Illness Is Killing Us **100**

**40** Pro Bodybuilders Choose Vegan **104**

**41** Pigs Are Smarter Than a Three-Year-Old Child **106**

**42** Chickens Like to Be Cuddled **109**

**43** Every Time You Buy Chicken, You Hurt a Farmer **111**

**44** Cows Love Classical Music **115**

**45** You Can Have Your Burger and Eat It, Too **117**

**46** There's No Need to Spend on Supplements **119**

**47** Beans Help You Live Longer **122**

**48** You Can Save Money **127**

**49** Plant Foods = Zero Cholesterol **130**

**50** Those Terrible Trans Fats Are Still Around **132**

**51** Type 2 Diabetes Is Not About Carbs. It's About Fat. **134**

**52** You Can Be Vegan*ish* **136**

**53** Because Babies! **139**

**54** Being Vegan Can Make You Happier **141**

**55** Crowding Out Food Is Easier Than Cutting Out Food **143**

**56** You Can Lower Your Body Fat **148**

**57** Good Genes Need Plants **150**

**58** Spent Dairy Cows Become Hamburgers and Dog Food **152**

**59** Meat Is the New Tobacco **154**

**60** The Meat Business Costs You Money **158**

**61** Pandemics Like COVID-19 Are Preventable **162**

**62** You Will Have Seriously Good Poops **165**

**63** Dogs and Cats Aren't the Only Loving Animals **167**

**64** It's Basic: Do unto Others **169**

**65** Wildlife Is Killed to Protect Animal Agriculture **170**

**66** You Could Ward Off Alzheimer's **172**

**67** Going Vegan Helps Prevent and Treat Arthritis **175**

**68** Vegan Is Sexy **177**

**69** #Chocolate **178**

**70** Animal Products Are Linked to Cancer **180**

**71** Fish Feel Pain **184**

**72** This Lifestyle Is an Ongoing Adventure **187**

*Acknowledgments* **188**

*Notes* **190**

*About the Authors* **200**

# Introduction

Hello, and welcome to our book. We think it's great that you're considering shifting from eating animals to eating plants, no matter how serious you are, and no matter what your timetable is.

Still, you might be thinking, "This is so out of my comfort zone . . . I don't know if I can do it." Check that. Both of us were once there, too.

Don't worry about it. Seriously. Just read, think, absorb, and see how you feel. There's no pressure. This is an exploration, and if you've got this book in your hands, you'll come to the conclusion that's right for you.

Neither of us grew up vegan. We both ended up here later in life, perhaps wishing it had been earlier, but grateful we got here at all.

## ABOUT US

*Hi, I'm Kathy.* I'm a southerner. I grew up in the town of Doraville, Georgia, population a little over eight thousand. While I was growing up, there was a steady stream of chicken-fried steak and collards with ham hock. Dad threw a steak on the grill on Sundays, and Mom loved to make bacon and eggs for my brothers and me. When I was a teenager, my idea of a healthy smoothie was whole-fat milk, fruit, and a raw egg. My friends and I regularly met for pizza and chicken wings, and on the nights at home in front of the TV, we all dug into a big box of vanilla ice cream. My point is: I ate plenty of animal food and never thought twice about it.

Food is so much about family and community, so these BBQs and burgers were a large part of my social life and overall sense of belonging. As I got older, I paid more attention to the news and began watching videos online. I gradually realized that maybe I wasn't making the healthiest food choices.

**I ate plenty of animal food and never thought twice about it.**

Then, about sixteen years ago, I was playing with my little dog and a light bulb went on in my brain: This animated ball of fur was no different from a pig, a goat, a chicken, or a cow. They're all playful and funny. If I loved my dog, I'd probably love any animal I got to know. Suddenly, it felt weird and disgusting to think about eating animals.

Considering how much I loved eating meat and dairy, this was an inconvenient awakening. I did not make the move overnight. I explored different foods and recipes, menus and restaurants, and over the course of about a year I became vegan. I researched the health implications of animal-based foods and found that by avoiding them I would be doing my body a great service, and that my energy and health would greatly improve. (It did.) And as a bonus, the science suggested I could live up to a decade longer by eating a plant-based diet.

I still love community and food culture. But now I'm all about tweaking traditional meals so that they're kinder to the body and easier on the environment and animals. That means holiday meals with vegan sausages and a plant-based holiday loaf rather than turkey or ham; Beyond Meat or Impossible Burgers instead of meat from a cow; and quinoa and kale rather than fish. I love salads, but only if there are warm, tasty morsels tossed in, such as blackened corn, cannellini beans, or falafel. I follow in the footsteps of my parents, who enjoyed cheese and crackers every day for happy hour, but I opt for almond or cashew cheese and hummus or guacamole instead of dairy. And on Friday nights, I like a good martini—up, dry, extra cold, with ice, and olives on the side.

I'm not a purist. I believe in progress rather than perfection. I believe in "crowding out" rather than "cutting out" so that the shift toward being healthy and kind is an easy one, rather than a white-knuckle effort. I believe that if we're given good information and friendly advice on how to apply it to our lives, it's our evolutionary impulse to move forward. I'm hoping we can all do just that.

*Hello. My name is Gene,* and I'm a meataholic. At least, I was. When I was growing up, I refused to eat vegetables. Ever. All I wanted was steak, burgers, and hot dogs. There was a small drawer in the kitchen table right in front of where I always sat for dinner. One night my mother smelled a strange odor and opened the drawer. To her horror, she found years of rotting vegetables that I had secretly slipped into the drawer so I could claim my plate was clean. I was immediately sent to my room and forced to eat spinach for the rest of my life. Well, the first part of that, yes. Not the second. I still refused to eat vegetables.

Veggies remained the bane of my existence until I started to live on my own, when I finally began adding carrots, broccoli, and even the occasional salad to my daily diet. They were cheaper and easier to cook than meat. Like Kathy, I became increasingly interested in health, and I read more and more about meat and its impact on health. I decided to start slow and become a pescatarian—that is, a person who avoids meat, but does eat fish. I thought I'd miss steak, pork, and chicken, but that didn't happen. Then, I decided to take it a step further and became vegetarian. I thought I'd miss fish, but that didn't happen. Finally, about a dozen years later, I met a vegan firefighter in Texas, Rip Esselstyn, with whom I eventually wrote three books. To write the first book, I figured it would make sense to at least *try* being vegan, even though I was still a total cheese-hound.

It stuck. (And although I missed cheese, I found out there were excellent nut cheeses on the market, and I've become something of a connoisseur.) And as I became more and more interested in our environment, I read about how animal-based foods are among the worst contributors to greenhouse gases. That clinched it.

Going vegan probably worked for me because, being a rather lazy person, I found the transition much easier than my carnivorous comrades told me it would be. I'd thought a plant-based diet would be dull and difficult. It wasn't. Every year more and more interesting non-animal-based products came on the market, more and more skilled chefs published cookbooks featuring plant-based meals, and eventually even some of those carnivores who told me they'd never give up meat became curious. "What's your reason for being vegan?" they'd ask.

And that's why I wanted to write this book, because for me, there isn't a single reason. There are dozens and dozens of reasons. You will soon read many of them. Believe it or not, there are plenty more. (You can find these extras on our Facebook page. Visit us and tell us your reasons.) And there are plenty of ways of doing it, too, from going cold Tofurky to just slowly eating more and more fruits and vegetables, until you've pushed animals off your plate entirely.

In fact, one of the best parts of going vegan is that all of a sudden a whole new world of food is available—not that it wasn't before, but like most nonvegans, I had limited my choices of plants to the basics: potatoes, spinach, apples, bananas, and so on. Now I have become fond of passion fruit, jackfruit, amaranth, artichokes, gar-

**Instead of limiting my diet, I grew it.**

lic scapes, and cherimoyas. I know the differences among white, green, and purple asparagus. I know how wonderful leeks can taste, I look forward to ramp season, and I even know what kohlrabi is—and I love it. In other words, my food choices became exciting, eclectic, and delicious. Instead of limiting my diet, I grew it.

# 01

# VEGANISM IS HAPPENING IN A VERY MAJOR WAY

I f you're already vegan, you're a trailblazer for an international trend that's growing larger every year. Less than a generation ago, veganism (and vegetarianism, for that matter) was beyond the fringe, considered just a dietary choice of a bunch of freaks, hippies, and health nuts (and a small number of forward-thinking doctors). Vegan restaurants, much less dairy-free milks, nut-based cheeses, and meatless burgers, were few and far between. Even as recently as 2014, only 1 percent of Americans identified as vegan.

Flash forward to 2019, which *The Economist* called "The Year of the Vegan." In the previous five years, the number of self-reported vegans has skyrocketed by 600 percent.[1] It has been mostly millennials leading the charge—about 15 percent say they're vegan (and even more say they're vegetarian). It's changing the way we eat, and even the way we celebrate. In mid-November 2018, according to Google Trends, "Vegan Thanksgiving" was the top diet-related search. And it's not just in the United States: Web searches in *any* language for vegan-related topics continue to reach all-time highs, with Australia, the UK, and New Zealand leading the way. If you seek an enchilada or pierogi on your next trip to Mexico or Poland, it may well be a bean or spinach version: 9 percent and 7 percent of these nations' population are vegan, respectively—at least fourteen million people combined.

The movement is putting its money where its mouth is: The Plant Based Foods Association reported 20 percent growth in US supermarket sales in 2018—the equivalent of more than $3 billion in containers of coconut milk yogurt, tempeh bacon, and the like. Michele Simon, the group's executive director, pointed out, "The plant-based foods industry has gone from being a relatively niche market to fully mainstream. . . . Plant-based meat and dairy alternatives are not just for vegetarians or vegans anymore." So, it's no surprise that traditional food giants worldwide have begun including their own plant-based options. Subway, Burger King, KFC, Taco Bell, Starbucks, and many others are now featuring vegan options that, in some cases, are outselling their meaty ones.[2]

In some countries, veganism isn't just becoming popular—it's becoming policy. The Canadian government's *Food Guide* emphasizes plant-based eating, favoring tofu and beans over meat. Health insurance giant Kaiser Permanente recommends a plant-based diet in its Nutritional Update for Physicians. Vegan meals are being served in cafeterias across Los Angeles's public school system.

There are many reasons for becoming vegan, but who wants to be left behind on the trail when the blazers are so far in front of you that you can barely see them anymore?

# 02

# COWS BURP AND FART = METHANE = CLIMATE CHANGE

Cows chew grass or grain. This makes them gassy, so they burp and fart. The gas they pass is called methane, which is a very powerful global warming gas with twenty-eight times the warming potential of carbon dioxide. While most people think that $CO_2$ is the bad boy of greenhouse gases, methane is far more potent in the short term because it is extremely adept at trapping the sun's heat. The oil and gas industry is certainly the top offender when it comes to producing methane, but livestock is also a dangerous culprit.

Cows may look sweet and innocent; their farts are anything but.

Cows are ruminants, meaning the bacteria in their four stomachs digest food by fermenting it. This produces a lot of methane, most of which is expelled when a cow burps and, to a lesser extent, farts. Now, the average cow passes around 150 to 265 pounds of methane per year,[3] so if you multiply that figure by about a billion and a half—that's the number of cows worldwide—you'll end up with . . . a lot of methane . . . and a lot of climate change.

If you eat less beef, that means fewer cows, which means less burping and farting, which means less methane, which means less climate change.

# IT'S CHEAPER AND
# BETTER THAN
# BUYING A TESLA

C ool Tesla, bro! It feels pretty sweet to shift into Ludicrous Mode and tear down the highway powered by zero-emission battery bliss. And if you can afford one, a Tesla or other electric vehicle (EV) is the best way to reduce your carbon footprint . . . Kinda. Sorta. Maybe. Not really.

It's true that if you are going to drive, EVs are hands down the best option. If everyone drove an EV instead of a gasoline-powered car, the world would be a much cleaner place. Unfortunately, for the time being, they are also too expensive for most people. But while a Tesla may be out of reach for most consumers, there's good news: Driving an EV is nowhere near the most important way to reduce your carbon footprint. You can do far more for the environment right in your kitchen.

Researchers from the University of California, Riverside, have found that the total greenhouse gas emissions associated with a single charbroiled hamburger is equal to driving an eighteen-wheeler for 143 miles.[4] Similarly, a study out of the University of Chicago confirmed that simply ditching the Standard American Diet is more effective at combating climate change than switching to a hybrid electric car.* All told, as a Loma Linda University study found, vegans generate about 42 percent fewer greenhouse gas emissions than meat-eaters.

If you think the tailpipe in your neighbor's Hummer is dirty, it's got nothing on the tailpipes of the world's 1.4 billion cattle raised for meat and dairy. While adorable, these walking, mooing greenhouse-gas factories are farting out enormous amounts of methane every single day (see page 8). And when you consider all the diesel-guzzling trucks required to transport cows from feedlots to slaughter, and the countless more refrigerated trucks used to transport meat to grocery stores and restaurants, your sexy new EV isn't going to help the earth as long as it's still bringing you to the McDonald's drive-through.

If you want to be a true environmental superstar, you can be vegan *and* drive an EV. (Tesla has even eliminated leather interior options.) Or, better yet, take public transportation. EVs are certainly the future, so, if you must drive, don't pull the plug on that shiny new Model 3 just yet. But if your main concern is reducing your carbon footprint while not breaking the bank, forget your garage and take a hard look at your kitchen.

---

*Going plant-based is a lot cheaper, too. Dried beans cost about $2 per pound. A base-level Toyota Prius costs $24,000—or 12,000 pounds of black beans. Mmmmm.

# SOY IS PROTECTIVE AGAINST BREAST CANCER (AND WON'T GIVE GUYS MAN BOOBS)

If you believe the hype, you might think that soy, a common protein source for vegans and vegetarians, is the devil's dose of poison and that consuming it causes men to grow boobs and women to get breast cancer.

Do not fear for your chest. Sadly, soy is maligned in large part because it is such a good alternative to meat and dairy. It's brimming with protein and chock-full of calcium and iron—and it's been constantly and totally vilified by the meat and dairy industries. ("Kill the competition before people figure out how good and cheap it is," you might imagine hearing corporate executives say as they direct their marketing minions.)

Here's the truth: Soy has been a staple food and drink for thousands of years, mostly in Asia, where, until the Western diet was recently introduced, there was pretty much no breast cancer. Or man boobs. Contrary to what disinformation campaigns about soy might have told you, "Epidemiological studies have found that soy protein may reduce the risk for cancers including breast, colon, and prostate," the Physicians Committee for Responsible Medicine explains. "Studies show that women who include soy products in their routine are less likely to develop breast cancer, compared with other women."[6]

The bottom line? Regular consumption of soy (meaning, you aren't downing a couple hundred bottles of soy milk in one sitting) has no adverse effects on women or men.

Let's break it down: For women, the concern about soy in terms of breast cancer is estrogen. Estrogen is a *growth* hormone, and it makes cancer cells grow and proliferate, just like fertilizer makes weeds grow like crazy. Estrogen = fertilizer. (That's why dairy—which is naturally full of estrogen, since cow's milk is breast milk meant to make a baby cow grow to be two thousand pounds—is bad news if you're worried about cancer.)

But estrogen, which is made by mammals like humans and cows, is different from *phyto*estrogen, which is found in plants, like soy. (*Phyto* means plant.) Phytoestrogen is similar in structure to estrogen, but it's a much smaller compound; it sneaks its way out in front of mammal estrogen to attach to the estrogen receptor in our bodies, kind of like a small plane zipping in front of a jumbo jet and hooking up to the jetway before the jumbo ever had a chance to land.

Phytoestrogen = small plane. Estrogen = jumbo jet. Jetway = receptor/pathway into your body. Small plane blocks big plane, so the bad stuff has less opportunity to venture into your body. That wily little plane *blocks* the estrogen, thus making

## HERE'S THE TRUTH:

Soy has been a staple
food and drink for
thousands of years,
mostly in Asia, where,
until the Western diet
was recently introduced,
there was pretty much
no breast cancer.

it cancer-protective! (The scientific words are anti-proliferative and anti-carcinogenic.) That's why you'll hear a lot of doctors actually *recommend* eating more soy after a breast cancer diagnosis, because the science shows that women who start consuming soy after diagnosis have a decreased risk of recurrence![7] Of course, the only thing better than to start eating soy after disease diagnosis is to eat it proactively early in life; studies show that early and generous soy consumption (like that of traditional Japanese diets) is protective and healthy. And the same mechanism that protects women from breast cancer also blocks estrogen from getting into a man's system; hence, less chance of man boobs than if he consumed no tofu at all.

There is debate about whether people with hypothyroidism should avoid soy products, as it may interfere with their medication. Here's what the Mayo Clinic has to say: "There's no evidence that people who have hypothyroidism should avoid soy completely. If you have hypothyroidism, take thyroid hormone replacement as directed by your doctor. Medication can be taken at any time that's best for you, and it's okay to take it on an empty stomach or with food—as long as you do the same thing every day. Generally, it's best to wait four hours after taking thyroid medication to consume any products that contain soy."[8] (As always, you should consult your doctor to develop a meal system that works best for your unique needs.)

Now let's celebrate what soy *does* do! It's a very high-quality protein that is easily assimilated by the body and has the ideal composition of amino acids, meaning that you don't have to balance it out with grains to make a complete protein. It's already perfect. It contains lots of fiber and is also a great source of magnesium, potassium, and iron.

If possible, opt for organic soy, because then you're getting it free of glyphosate (the active ingredient in popular herbicides), GMOs, and whatever else crops are cultivated with when they come from big corporate farms. People who think they have allergies to soy may just be reacting to the chemicals it's been sprayed with, so eating organic can make a difference.

And by the way, we're not advocating that you should eat as much soy as possible, only that you need not be worried about eating it. There are plenty of other great protein-rich vegan foods you can enjoy, of which soy is just one healthy and delicious option!

**FOOD FACT:** First domesticated in China around 1100 BCE, soybeans were not just for food. The Chinese have been using moldy soybean curds to treat skin infections for many thousands of years.

**FACT:**

There's nothing gross about an oat milk latte or coconut ice cream.

# COW'S MILK IS
# KIND OF GROSS

Here's an idyllic scene: The kindly milk-man deposits a carton of fresh milk in lovely glass bottles on your doorstep. The milk is from the local dairy farm, where the cows graze lazily in lush, green fields; it's creamy and delicious and is a product of only the happiest cows. Drinking this lovely product makes you strong and healthy. Everyone wins! It's a perfect picture of paradise.

Except it's not paradise, dairy milk isn't perfect, and it certainly doesn't come from the happiest cows. On modern dairy farms, cows are both genetically and chemically manipulated to produce a lot of milk. Like, a *scary* amount of milk. Thirty years ago, the average dairy cow produced a little over thirteen thousand pounds of milk per year. More recently, she squeezes out more than twenty-one thousand pounds—an increase of 61 percent.[9] This is the result of the dairy industry selectively breeding cows to produce huge amounts of milk, all while injecting them with a cocktail of antibiotics and hormones to make them produce even more. This is true even for many smaller-scale farms. In order for dairy farmers to remain competitive in such a consolidated industry, their cows have to produce as much milk as chemically possible.

Plenty of people assume that female cows always produce milk, but like humans, cows only produce milk after they give birth. If she's not producing milk, the cow is not profitable for the farm. For this reason, the vast majority of dairy cows undergo artificial insemination soon after they stop producing milk. (Quite literally, a worker holding a load of bull sperm inserts their arm up a cow's vagina to impregnate her.) Female calves eventually become dairy cows, too, and because males can't produce milk, they are typically locked up in crates, slaughtered, and sold as veal.

The cows are milked relentlessly for ten months until their milk production decreases, and then they are artificially impregnated once again. Because of the stress associated with producing such extreme amounts of milk, dairy cows often suffer from a condition called mastitis, a painful and often fatal (for cows) inflammation of the mammary glands and udder tissue. In response, the cow's immune system pumps out somatic cells, which are composed largely of inflammatory immune cells that form pus. Mastitis is so common—the USDA reports that one in six dairy cows suffer from it—that there are approximately 1,120,000 somatic cells per *spoonful* of cow's milk.[10] In case you missed it: That's pus that comes along with the milk.

Cows can normally live twenty years or longer. Dairy cows rarely reach their sixth birthday. (For more about the plight of dairy cows, see page 152.)

So, how about sticking to plant-based milks? There's nothing gross about an oat milk latte or coconut ice cream.

# YOUR SKIN WILL LOOK AMAZING

D on't you just *love* waking up the morning of a presentation, wedding, or hot date with a big beautiful pimple on your nose? And didn't you think that your acne would clear up after you graduated high school? Maybe after college? Certainly by age thirty??

It could be your diet's fault.

And you aren't alone.

It turns out that people who eat a lot of dairy (cheese, yogurt, milk, and so on) have a higher propensity to break out. In a study published in the *Archives of Dermatology*, researchers following 1,300 predominantly plant-based people in New Guinea and remote regions of Paraguay could not diagnose a single pimple over two years.[11]

What's going on here? The culprit can be dairy itself, yes, but it's also what goes into dairy products, too. Dairy cows are given

**People who eat a lot of dairy have a higher propensity to break out.**

artificial hormones and antibiotics that boost milk production—chemicals that can trigger acne breakouts when consumed by humans. Even the hormones naturally found in cow's milk can exacerbate acne, so while switching to organic dairy products may improve the situation, it won't make your skin glow.

More proof: Harvard University researchers followed six thousand girls ages nine to fifteen for several years to see if there was a link between diet and skin appearance. Sure enough, the study found a "positive association between intake of milk and acne,"[12] and the results were confirmed in a subsequent study involving teenage boys. Other studies suggest that excess calories, added sugars, and meat can also affect protein signaling, making your body pump out more acne-causing oil and sebum.

So, say you'll cut out the animal products to clear up your acne—excellent, but don't stop there! Fruits and vegetables are loaded with antioxidants, which decrease inflammation and neutralize harmful free radicals—unstable atoms that can damage cells, cause disease, and prematurely age the body inside and out. For the supplest, most wrinkle-free skin, eat the rainbow of naturally colorful plants. Think fresh plump tomatoes, sweet potatoes, yellow bell peppers, blueberries, spinach, and beets. Fruits and vegetables are also loaded with carotenoids, which have been proven to promote a glowing skin tone.

The conclusion? If you want better skin, spend some more time in the produce aisle!

# FIBER IS YOUR
# BODY'S BITCH

Vegans, assuming they're not consuming mostly processed foods, eat high-fiber diets. Fiber is a kind of skeleton for plants, helping them maintain their shape and structure. When you eat unprocessed plant foods, you end up crunching down on a lot of it. The fiber from fruits, veggies, grains, nuts, and beans then mixes with the liquid in your gut to create a gel-like substance. As you digest your food, that gel slows the absorption of sugars and the subsequent release of insulin into the bloodstream. At the same time, it pushes against the stretch receptors in your stomach, telling your brain you've eaten enough. The result is that you feel full—and your energy remains steady and strong because of the slowed release of blood sugar.

Once in your body, fiber acts like a scrub brush pushing through your colon, grabbing stuff from inside the nooks and crannies in your 25-foot-long intestinal tract, and helping to usher it all out your back end, effectively getting rid of any old gunk, including carcinogens and other waste, that might otherwise cause a problem if left in your system. One thing fiber does leave behind: a healthy gut biome. It feeds the good bacteria in your belly that help regulate inflammation and immune function.

More and more research on fiber confirms that it has numerous other health benefits, such as lowering your cholesterol levels, as well as lowering your risk of diabetes, heart disease, and several types of cancer, meaning that the more fiber you eat, the more likely you are to live longer. Eating fiber is also one of the best ways to achieve a healthy weight. And, you'll have more regular, normal bowel movements, while reducing the risk of hemorrhoids.

**Only plants have fiber. Meat, dairy, and eggs have none.**

So, eat fiber. As much as possible. For men, that means about 40 grams a day, and for women, about 25 grams (about 20 percent less if you're over 50). And remember to drink lots and lots of water—fiber works best when it absorbs water.

Only plants have fiber. Meat, dairy, and eggs have none.

# DAIRY DOESN'T DO
# A BODY GOOD

D o you have any of the following symptoms after eating dairy: bloating, excessive farting, burping or belching, pain, cramping, a belly that looks nine months pregnant, or a slight feeling that your stomach might just simply explode? If so, there's a good chance you are lactose intolerant, just like 65 percent of the global population.[13] A lot of people are misdiagnosed with IBS (irritable bowel syndrome) when what they are really experiencing is a genetic inability to digest cheese or milk.

Lactose intolerance is the most common genetic deficiency worldwide, and it comes from not having enough lactase (an enzyme meant to break down milk sugar) in your system to digest the lactose (sugar) from milk. So if you're among the 65 percent, the undigested lactose you ingest when indulging in dairy causes inflammation, bringing massive amounts of water into your small intestine and colon, which then could lead to watery diarrhea and major bloat. Bacteria in your colon finally metabolize the undigested lactose, and you get some mighty malodourous fermentation churning away down there, which eventually escapes your body as smelly gas.

People who are lactose intolerant often think there is something wrong with them and treat it like a medical condition. But when you consider that the majority of the world's population can't digest dairy, it's worth thinking of lactose intolerance as normal. It makes sense: Why should we be able to properly digest the milk of other animals? Biologically speaking, we are not intended to drink dairy (the fluid of a lactating animal that is designed by nature for her baby).

Some people are mildly lactose intolerant, which means they experience only mild nausea, gas, or general discomfort. Humans are remarkable animals who can adapt to and live with regular pain, but why not figure out if you have lactose intolerance and can do away with that stomachache? Just give up dairy 100 percent for at least a month. Check labels to make sure it's not hiding in your salad dressing, cookies, and other sneaky places, because food manufacturers love putting dairy everywhere. Look for ingredients like casein and its derivatives (caseinate, for example), lactate, curds, ghee, and whey. Try oat, almond, hemp, coconut, rice, or soy milk instead of cow's milk, and you'll very likely get a flatter belly and a whole lot less gas. And if you're a cheese freak, look for the ton of nondairy cheeses in the market now. Same for ice cream, yogurt, and even ranch or blue-cheese dressing.

Note: Lactose intolerance is different from "dairy sensitivity." Dairy sensitivity means that you essentially have an allergic reaction to the cow's milk proteins, and that can lead to such issues as eczema, serious sinus problems, inflammatory bowel disease, and damage to the gastrointestinal lining. The solution to both conditions is the same, however: Don't consume dairy.

Check out Switch4Good.org to find out more.

# ANTIBIOTIC
# RESISTANCE
# IS NO JOKE

S cared of cancer? You should be. It's a terrifying disease. But are you scared of antibiotic-resistant infections, too? Again, you should be, because these infections kill more people per year than breast and prostate cancer combined.

Yet with all the research and money that goes into fighting cancer, we are spending very little time and money figuring out why antibiotics, once considered wonder drugs that would end disease, aren't working as well as they used to. Could the "end of antibiotics" be near?[14] Some scientists think so, which means that they can imagine a new breed of infections that will prove impervious to antibiotics. Imagine a bladder infection, strep throat, or an infected cut on your big toe that could spread throughout your body unchecked, shut down your organs, and kill you. How? Because germs, exposed to so many antibiotics, have evolved and mutated to the point that the drugs are much less effective—and, increasingly, entirely ineffective.[15] Bacteria are one-celled organisms, but they're smarter than you think: Just like us, they want to live, so they've been busy adapting to hide from, trick, and, above all, resist those once-lethal drugs. Our antibiotics didn't quite kill off *all* those bacteria, and now those bacteria are becoming unstoppable.

What's this got to do with veganism? The problem stems in part from the over-prescription of antibiotics (too many nervous parents give their toddlers a dose of antibiotics at the first sign of a sniffle, for example). But the problem extends far beyond the doctor's office and onto factory farms, which are simply filthy places. Stressed-out animals are packed into cramped enclosures, living in each other's poop and muck, making them vulnerable to sickness. To prevent livestock from dying before they reach slaughter weight, animal handlers regularly dose their animals with all kinds of powerful antibiotics and medicines—many of them the same as those that humans use. Moreover, because antibiotics make animals grow faster (meaning they can be sent to the slaughterhouse quicker), farmers routinely pump *healthy* cows, chickens, and pigs full of them, too.

There's your exposure: Antibiotics are fed to animals. Animals are slaughtered. And with every bite of hot dog, cheeseburger, steak, and other animal products you eat, you are microdosing yourself with the antibiotics that were in their systems—and, over time, contributing to the problem of antibiotic resistance.

**PHARMACEUTICAL FACT:** Approximately 70 percent of all medically important antibiotics in the United States are used on farm animals.[16]

# DUDE,
# YOUR ERECTIONS
# *#BETTERLONGER*

What makes for a really good erection? Excellent blood flow. When men become aroused, blood flows readily into the penis and engorges it. When blood flow is restricted, it tends to be restricted *everywhere*, whether it's the heart or the penis. As the Cleveland Clinic explains, "There is a very strong link between erectile dysfunction and heart disease. Several studies have shown that if a man has ED, he has a greater risk of having heart disease."[17] Similarly, a study published in the *Journal of Urology* found that 68 percent of men with high blood pressure also had some degree of erectile dysfunction.[18]

What's one of the best ways to make sure that your blood is flowing? Eat the same plant-strong diet you would eat to heal your heart. Medical evidence indicates that the saturated fat in meat and dairy clogs up the arteries going to *all* organs.

A recent study of Canadian men with diabetes reported that risk of erectile dysfunction was 10 percent lower with every daily serving of fruits and/or vegetables. In other words, an apple a day keeps the Viagra away.

# GALS,
# YOUR CLITORIS
# #ORGASMS

Our friend Jane Esselstyn is a nurse, author, researcher, married mother of three, and middle school sex-ed teacher—which is why we listen to her when she talks about sex. The following are her comments:

Just as blood flow is essential for an erection, (see reason 10, opposite), it also helps women to achieve sexual readiness via lubrication. Front and center in this blood-flow discussion is the clitoris, the little bundle of eight thousand nerves south of the pubic bone and just ahead of the vaginal urethral opening. Yet the clitoris is just the beginning. When a woman is aroused, after the clitoris engorges with blood, tissues inside the pelvis engorge as well. These tissues, called the crura and the corpus cavernosa, line both sides of the vaginal space in winglike formation. Like the engorge-able tissue found in the shaft of the penis, the crura and the corpus cavernosa fill with blood; as they do, they lasso around the vaginal space and cause deeper arousal.

To recap: Major food source high in the saturated fats that limit blood flow to sexual organs = meat. Major food source low in saturated fats, which enhances blood flow to sexual organs = vegetables.

# MOST FISH
# ARE POLLUTED
# BY MERCURY
# AND PLASTIC

Hankering for halibut? Yearning for yellowtail? Craving cod? You might want to dream again unless you enjoy meals featuring toxic compounds and vermin.

Let's start with mercury, a silvery-white element that is liquid at room temperature. The World Health Organization considers mercury one of the top ten "chemicals of major public health concern"—and yet it's widely found in fish. Mercury can harm the central nervous system and can cause developmental disabilities in babies born to mothers with high levels of the chemical in their body. Mercury finds its way into fish from several sources. When coal and other fossil fuels are burned, mercury-containing emissions are carried into the ocean by rain. Mercury from household and industrial waste finds its way into soil and then ground water. Naturally occurring bacteria convert it into a compound called methylmercury, which gets eaten by plankton, who are then eaten by small fish, who are then eaten by bigger fish. As the methylmercury moves up the food chain, it becomes more concentrated.

It gets worse. Mercury isn't the only contaminant in fish, who contain a whole bouillabaisse of toxic chemicals, including pesticides, dioxin, and PCBs from industrial, farm, and stormwater runoff that wash into waterways, where fish absorb them. All of these pollutants can build up in your body over time and can take years to eliminate.

Sadly, pollutants are everywhere: In 2009 the US Environmental Protection Agency conducted a study of freshwater fish contamination in five hundred lakes and reservoirs across all states. They found mercury and PCBs in all of them.[19] *All* of them. Moreover, a 2016 global analysis of seafood by the Scripps Institution of Oceanography found that all types of the world's ocean fish contain toxic chemicals known as persistent organic pollutants (POPs) in varying levels.[20] *All* of them.

> **Methylmercury becomes more concentrated as it moves up the food chain.**

Still want to risk it for the spicy dragon roll? How do you feel about spicy parasite roll? Raw fish entrees like sushi and sashimi are prone to harbor the likes of tapeworms or a nematode called *Anisakis*, nicknamed the herring worm. These creatures' eggs are excreted via human or sea animal feces and hatch in water. Their larvae get eaten by crustaceans, who are then eaten by fish. As the worms grow, their presence can lead to symptoms including abdominal cramps, severe diarrhea, and vomiting till the parasite is removed. Pass the avocado-and-cucumber roll, please!

# 13

# HEALTHY FATS COME FROM NUTS, SEEDS, AND AVOCADOS

Not from marbled steak, pork ribs, or chicken fingers. Contrary to the "low-fat" diet fad of the 1990s, we *do* need fat in our diets, and quite a bit: up to 30 percent of our daily calories. Fat is important for cell growth, protecting your organs, making hormones, and even keeping you warm.

But all fats are not created equal. Animal fat contains mostly saturated and trans fat, the types that jack up your "L-for-lethal" LDL cholesterol and cause plaque to accumulate in, harden, and then block your arteries so blood can't flow freely. That's called atherosclerosis, and it's long been linked to cardiovascular disease including heart attack and stroke. Too much saturated fat can also lead to insulin resistance, the precursor to diabetes.

The American Heart Association recommends replacing most saturated fat—like that in butter and bacon—with healthier mono- and polyunsaturated fats. Where do you get that? Plant foods. They provide essential fatty acids, so called because your body can't make them and they're vital for things like energy storage and absorbing vitamins. Your best sources of healthy fats are nuts, seeds, avocados (and guacamole!), olives, certain cold-pressed vegetable oils such as extra-virgin olive oil and flaxseed, pistachios, pumpkin seeds, and don't forget peanut butter!

All of these are rich in omega-3 and omega-6 fatty acids, which are great for your brain, your immune system, and your blood pressure. And they're delicious and filling—and easy to snack on and toss into salads and put on sandwiches. Don't go too bonkers on the oils, though—they are high in calories.

**FAT IS IMPORTANT:**

It helps with cell growth, protecting your organs, making hormones, and even keeping you warm. But all fats are not created equal.

# WE CAN SOLVE
# WORLD HUNGER

One in nine people around the world goes to bed hungry every night. Think about what that's like: You can't focus on work or relationships. You don't have the energy to take care of business or your family. You start feeling run down and desperate, and your health suffers. Well, over eight hundred million people feel that way every single day of their lives.

Here's the crazy part: There are enough resources—enough food—to feed everyone who needs it. But sadly, a lot of the food that could go to humans, such as corn, wheat, and soy, goes to livestock instead. The animals we eat—cows, pigs, chickens, turkeys, lambs—also have to eat. And they have to eat a lot more calories in feed than they turn into meat, because, like humans, they burn calories just by breathing, moving, pooping, and so on. In fact, cycling grains and legumes through animals to produce meat wastes at least 90 percent of the caloric input. That's like throwing 90 percent of perfectly good food in the garbage when it could have gone to feeding hungry people! That's wasteful with a capital *W*.

When you think of the billions of animals on this planet who are raised and killed for food each year, you might scratch your head and wonder why we have this inefficient system of producing calories. (Hint: It only makes sense if you're in the meat biz.)

We could simply cut out the middleman—or, in this case, the middlecow—and give the food to the global poor. Instead, the valuable and nutritious corn, wheat, and soy is shipped to factory farms to feed animals who are being fattened up for slaughter. The bottom line is that as long as the animal agriculture industry is willing to pay more for the grain used to feed their animals than developing nations can afford for the same food, the global poor will remain hungry.

> **We could simply cut out the middleman … and give the food to the global poor.**

The good news is that we're already producing enough food worldwide to feed everyone in the world. In fact, according to researchers from Lancaster University, we're already producing enough food to feed the world's projected 9.7 billion population in 2050.

The only thing we have to do, according to the study? "[Replace] most meat and dairy with plant-based alternatives."[21] It's as simple as that.

# 15

# YOU COULD BE THE NEXT GANDHI, DA VINCI, OR TOLSTOY

Being committed to veganism was pretty difficult before the mid-twentieth century: Oat milk wasn't available at your local market, and the Beyond Burger wasn't sold at the local burger joint. And yet throughout history, numerous legendary figures were known to avoid meat, including Pythagoras (the first vegetarian on record), Buddha, George Bernard Shaw, and many, many more. Even St. Francis, who we'd like to imagine was so fond of animals that he chose not to eat them.

Today, being vegan is easy. Some people do it for health, some for the environment, and some for the animals, but the number of well-known vegans—from professional athletes to politicians to musicians to prizewinning authors and actors—grows every month, meaning that everyday vegans are in great company. Just to name a few: Oscar-winning actors Jessica Chastain and Joaquin Phoenix (vegan since childhood); Woody Harrelson (raw vegan for decades); and Spidey Tobey Maguire.

Musicians Madonna, Joan Jett, and Stevie Wonder also sing the praises of a plant-based diet.

Plant-powered politicians campaigning for eating less meat include New Jersey Senator Cory Booker, former Representative Dennis Kucinich, and Vice President Al Gore. Elite athletes also stay strong on predominantly vegan diets, including NFL quarterback and social justice activist Colin Kaepernick, tennis legends Venus and Serena Williams, and former NFL defensive lineman David Carter (aka The 300-Pound Vegan). MMA fighter Mac Danzig has been vegan for over a decade, and so has ultramarathon record holder Scott Jurek. Even former Ben & Jerry's–endorsing Olympic snowboarder Hannah Teter now endorses veganism.

Meat-shunning stars are using their platforms to share their passion and educate others: Former NBA star John Salley has a website exclusively devoted to vegan tips. *The Big Bang Theory*'s Mayim Bialik has a vegan cookbook. *Clueless* star Alicia Silverstone has several books in the vegan lifestyle category. Oscar winner Natalie Portman narrated a YouTube video, "9 Things Vegans Are Tired of Hearing," and co-produced the factory-farming documentary *Eating Animals*. Ellen DeGeneres and Portia DiRossi had a vegan wedding and continue to advocate for eating more vegan food. And, of course, Pamela Anderson famously posed naked for PETA ads.

When you become vegan, you are breaking bread with some of the most interesting people around.

**FANTASTIC FACT:** Mary Shelley, author of *Frankenstein*, was vegetarian. So was Frankenstein's monster.

# 16

# THE KETO DIET
# SHORTENS
# YOUR LIFE

The ketogenic, or "keto," diet is one of those fads that sounds new and exciting, but isn't. It's just a more extreme version of the low-carb Atkins diet of a half-century ago, which in its time was slammed as everything from "bizarre" to "dangerous" before being officially condemned by the American Medical Association.

Here's how keto works: Normally, you get your energy from stored blood sugar supplied by the carbohydrates you eat. If no carbs are available, your body switches to burning fat for fuel, a process called ketosis. Ketosis prompts rapid weight loss. Thus, the keto diet nixes all but about 30 grams of carbs from your meals (5 percent of calories) and replaces them with animal fat and protein. Think bun-less bacon cheeseburgers—all day, every day. No bread. No bananas. No natural sugars.

The keto diet was originally designed to treat epilepsy in children. It's also a way for very obese people under a doctor's care to lose pounds quickly. As a lifestyle for otherwise healthy people, though, it's a recipe for disaster.

For starters, it's not balanced. Humans need plenty of carbohydrates: The Institute of Medicine recommends we get 45 percent to 65 percent of our daily calories from them.[22] That doesn't mean Krispy Kremes, but the kind of complex carbs you can find only in plants: vegetables, fruits, beans and legumes, and whole grains. Among other things, carbs from veggies and fruits supply almost all the essential vitamins and minerals our body needs. And eating plants is the *only* way to obtain the fiber your gut and colon require to function properly. Not to mention disease-fighting phyto-nutrients, including vitamin C and flavonoids.

The loads of saturated fat and protein in the keto diet are not healthy either. Among other things, diets high in animal foods put you at risk for diabetes and heart disease. All that fat leaks into your bloodstream, causing inflammation and oxidative stress (the over-abundance of harmful free radicals). This in turn can lead to insulin resistance. Low-carb diets not only impair your arteries' func-tionality and gum up blood flow to the heart but also are linked to a shorter life span. According to a mas-sive study reported in *The Lancet* involving more than fifteen thousand peo-ple over twenty-five years, "Low-carb diets that replace carbohydrates with protein or fat are gaining widespread popularity as a health and weight-loss strategy. However, our data suggests that animal-based low-carbohydrate diets, which are prevalent in North America and Europe,

**Diets high in animal foods put you at risk for diabetes and heart disease.**

might be associated with shorter overall life span and should be discouraged."[23]

But wait, there's more: A study published by the American Heart Association found that people who eat low-carb, high-animal-protein diets might increase their risk of heart failure by 43 percent—and by nearly 49 percent when much of that protein comes from dairy.[24] Even if you get lucky and avoid a heart attack or stroke, you might not feel so hot on a keto diet. Side effects may include fatigue, constipation, headaches, indigestion, and bad breath.[†]

Ultimately, keto isn't sustainable. Why drown in grease and pine for potatoes when you can lose, maintain, or gain weight (depending on what you want), fulfill your nutritional needs, and eat delicious food on a whole-food vegan diet?

---

† And very smelly farts (see page 125).

# IRON IS NECESSARY.
# BUT IT TAKES PLANTS
# TO GET IT RIGHT.

I ron does a body good. Without it, humans could not exist. We need it to make DNA, our genetic blueprint; hemoglobin, which brings oxygen to all parts of the body; and myoglobin, which stores oxygen in our muscles that we use whenever we move. But you *can* get too much of a good thing, which is why the recommended upper limit is 45 milligrams of iron per day (the recommended daily allowance for adults is less than half that).

Fortunately, your body has a natural ability to absorb just the right amount of iron, as long as it is *nonheme* iron—the type found primarily in plant foods. On the other hand, the body quickly processes *heme* iron, which is found only in meat, poultry, and seafood, without any way to modulate or remove it. Instead, the body shuttles the extra heme iron into a protein called ferritin, which acts like a storage tank. When the "tank" gets too full, the ferritin and iron change into a rustlike substance called hemosiderin, which can build up in your organs.

"Free" heme iron creates oxidative stress, which is basically an imbalance between free radicals and antioxidants. This can trigger inflammation and cause cell and tissue damage, increasing your

## JUST RIGHT:

Your body has a natural ability to absorb just the right amount of iron, as long as it is *nonheme* iron—the type found primarily in plant foods.

chances of developing arthritis, cardiovascular conditions like high blood pressure, stroke, and heart disease; cancer; type 2 diabetes; Parkinson's disease; Alzheimer's disease; and metabolic syndrome. It also speeds up the aging (aka dying) process.

So, how to make sure you get enough iron without going overboard? You guessed it: a whole-food, plant-based diet. You can get plenty of nonheme iron from veggies and fruits including dark leafy greens, tofu, beans and legumes, whole grains, nuts and seeds, skin-on potatoes, molasses, and raisins, among other foods. Not only that: Chemicals in plants called phytates seem to help suppress the free radicals that heme iron creates and have been found to help reduce dangerous levels of iron in the body.

# WE AREN'T
# LIONS

Lions aren't just kings; they are also killers—they have daggerlike teeth and claws meant to maim. A female lion thrusts her powerful legs and overtakes her prey with speed and precision. She stalks, she pounces, and she gnashes into the back of a wounded animal's neck until it dies. The lion salivates at the carcass and then digs into her feast. Her jaws are so powerful they can crush bone, but, as with other pure carnivores, they only move up and down in a chomping way, which means she has to tear out chunks of flesh and swallow them whole. She has extremely acidic digestive juices in her stomach that kill any bacteria from the meat she's eating, and her short, smooth colon zips the waste quickly through her system as if it were a garbage chute. In short, these are the actions of an animal who is biologically designed to eat meat.

**"Our anterior teeth are not suited for tearing flesh or hide."**

Humans, on the other hand, see a wounded animal and feel a pang of sympathy. Most of us are repulsed to see a dead, bloodied carcass. We have soft fingernails, and molars that grind by moving side to side as well as up and down, so we can chew our fibrous (plant) food. We have weak stomach acid, meaning that raw, rotting meat can kill us. And we have a very long, windy, notched intestinal tract allowing for more time to break down fiber. Rotting meat can get stuck in the notches, allowing bacteria to flourish and make us sick.

Anthropologist Dr. Richard Leakey says it this way: "You can't tear flesh by hand, you can't tear hide by hand. Our anterior teeth are not suited for tearing flesh or hide. We don't have large canine teeth, and we wouldn't have been able to deal with food sources that require those large canines."[25]

So if your friends say, "Humans are meant to eat meat!," you can tell them that the exact opposite is true. Sure, we're omnivores in that we can eat just about anything and survive, but our physical and emotional systems are ideally suited for food grown in the ground or on trees and peacefully harvested.

# EGGS ARE NOT
# INCREDIBLE
# OR EDIBLE

Many people, when asked why they eat eggs, will say, "Because they're a good source of protein." But eggs *don't* have an especially large amount of protein—about 3 grams in the yolk and 3 grams in the white. Why not instead eat a cup of cooked lentils, which boasts 17 grams of protein while containing a healthy dose of fiber, folate, and other nutrients?

But before we go further into the egg's problems, here's a little unappetizing truth that you might want to consider: Eggs come out of a hen's cloaca, which is a combination of an anus, vagina, and urinary tract, all in one cavity. So, if you eat eggs, you're essentially eating the menstruation of a chicken, which happened to come out of her prolapsed asshole. Still sound good?

Back to the dietary stuff: Here are a few little issues with the not-so-incredible egg:

- One egg has about as much cholesterol (180 mg) as an 8-ounce steak. Dietary cholesterol— meaning, the cholesterol you get from food rather than what your body produces naturally— raises your risk of heart disease or stroke.

One population study of nearly 30,000 people found that for every daily 300-mg dose of dietary cholesterol, a person's risk of developing cardiovascular disease increased by 17 percent.[26] According to a 2019 study published in *JAMA* (*the Journal of the American Medical Association*), for each extra half egg eaten per day (totaling three or four more eggs per week), a person's cardiovascular disease risk went up by 6 percent, and his or her risk of early death increased by 8 percent.[27]

- Women who eat five eggs a week may significantly increase their chances of getting breast cancer, likely because cholesterol may play a role in the development and progression of breast cancer.[28]

- Eating one to two eggs per week may increase someone's risk of colon cancer by 19 percent compared with those who eat barely any, while someone who eats three or more eggs per week may see a 71 percent increased risk.[29]

- Men who eat an average of 2.5 eggs per week increase their risk of advanced and fatal forms of prostate cancer by 81 percent. Why? In addition to the cholesterol, eggs have a lot of choline, which may turn toxic in the digestive system, increasing prostate cancer risk. Remember that eggs are not only found in a morning scramble, but also in most baked goods, dressings, and many sauces, making it fairly easy to surpass that 2.5 average.[30]

- Eggs are often contaminated with *Salmonella*, which can make you wicked sick and even die.

- Egg whites are trouble, too, because they are a very concentrated source of animal protein, which can lead to kidney disease, kidney stones, and certain cancers.

So, don't skip breakfast. Just skip the eggs, lower your risks of a whole lot of problems, and eliminate some serious nastiness. What better way to start your morning?

**FUN FACT:** According to the CDC, protein deficiency in America is very rare. In fact, it's so rare that almost no one outside of a few specialists and spelling bee champs knows the word for protein malnutrition. In case you're curious, the word for protein malnourishment is *kwashiorkor*.

# GO FISH.
# NO FISH.

D o you like the taste of fresh-caught grilled fish? Or perhaps you prefer sushi, a nice shrimp cocktail, or ceviche? Well, enjoy them now if you must, since it's likely that your children or grandchildren will never get a chance to know what any of these ocean animals taste like.

Scary fact number ten gazillion: According to the World Wildlife Federation, the world's oceans may well be empty of fish by the year 2048 because of overfishing.[31] Other studies estimate that 70 percent of the global fish population is fully used, overused, or in crisis.[32]

What's happening?

We are running out of fish.

We don't know precisely how many individual fish are caught (they are measured by the ton), but the commercial fishing industry captures somewhere between one and three trillion fish per year. Yes, that's *trillion* with a *T*! This isn't rocket science: If you take three trillion fish out of the water every single year, they simply can't repopulate fast enough to keep up.

> **"Overfishing can impact entire ecosystems."**

Fishing techniques also contribute to this decimation. Forget the romantic image of a guy on a little boat with a fishing rod. Forget the heroic struggles of *The Old Man and the Sea*. Instead, think about vast industrial nets scooping up everything they can possibly collect, whether or not the resulting catches can be sold. How much of the dead or dying netted fish, known as bycatch, are then discarded back into the sea? About forty-two million tons a year.[33] All told, some 40 percent of all fish caught worldwide are unintentional bycatch (and don't forget the three hundred thousand whales, dolphins, and porpoises that are killed by fishing nets every year, not to mention the sharks, turtles, starfish, sponges, and hundreds of thousands of diving seabirds that become tangled in nets). This demolition doesn't happen just in the oceans. Fresh waters are also suffering from overfishing. Just one example: In the 1980s, the blue walleye population in the Great Lakes was overfished to complete extinction.

Equally alarming, plunging fish populations create ripple effects throughout the entire marine ecosystem, disrupting age-old predator–prey relationships. For example, a decline in pollack in western Alaska has caused a 90 percent decline in Steller's sea lions, who eat these fish but are now listed as endangered. And because of the decrease in sea lions, who are orcas' primary prey, orcas have been eating more sea otters. As a result, sea otter populations have declined rapidly since 1990. According to the World Wide Fund for Nature (aka the WWF, an organization that knows how to fight, as it won a multiyear battle with the World Wrestling Federation over the use of those initials), "Overfishing can impact entire ecosystems. . . .

When too many fish are taken out of the ocean, it creates an imbalance that can erode the food web and lead to a loss of other important marine life, including vulnerable species like sea turtles and corals."[34]

The good news? Fish stocks can recover if ecosystems are properly protected. Boris Worm, a marine conservationist and professor of biology at Dalhousie University in Halifax, Canada, led a 2006 study that discovered that inside forty-four protected areas studied, "Species came back more quickly than people anticipated—in three or five or 10 years."[35]

If we stop eating fish, we can save the oceanic world.

**FRACTIOUS FACT:** It's not just fish and other animals who are suffering. As large fishing vessels ply increasingly overfished seas, international conflicts are becoming more common. Scottish fishermen have attacked Russian trawlers. Russians have attacked Japanese vessels in the northwest Pacific. Norwegian patrols have shredded Icelandic nets in the Arctic. Their respective crews even exchanged gunfire. The United Nations has reported a sharp increase in piracy and armed robbery directed toward ships, many of them fishing vessels.

# FARMED FISH ARE
# NOT GOING TO
# SAVE WILD FISH

Why do we need to worry about catching wild fish in the ocean when we can just farm fish ourselves in controlled environments?

Unfortunately, fish farms are not the answer. For one, the most commonly farmed fish, including salmon, halibut, and cod, are fed fish taken from the oceans, thus furthering overextraction: Producing just one pound of edible food from captive fish requires three to four pounds of wild fish.

There's more: Farmed fish are an environmental disaster because they deplete natural resources. Fish reared in artificial ponds require enormous amounts of water to replenish oxygen and remove waste products. Most farmed fish, though, are raised in cages anchored to the sea floor. This might seem sustainable since existing bodies of water are used. However, the incredible amount of waste generated by farmed fish spills out from nets into open ocean, polluting fragile habitats with antibiotics and other harmful chemicals that the captive fish were doused with. Sometimes farmed fish escape their cages and breed with wild fish, weakening critical genetic traits for future generations.

Numerous studies have shown that some farmed fish, especially salmon, are rife with cancer-causing compounds such as polychlorinated biphenyls (PCBs), industrial chemicals that were manufactured from 1929 until 1979. According to a recent study commissioned by the Environmental Working Group, seven of ten farmed salmon purchased at grocery stores in Washington, DC, San Francisco, and Portland, Oregon, were contaminated with PCBs at levels that raise health concerns.[36]

Fish farming—which is essentially factory farming conducted in water—also requires a good deal of viable land that might otherwise be used for forests or crops. On top of all this, it's a terrible life for the fish themselves. The farm makes the most money by packing thousands and thousands of fish into troughs or cages, allowing each one barely enough space to breathe, no less swim. These conditions lead to disease, from viral and fungal infections to parasites. What happens when animals get diseases? We give them as many antibiotics as we can. Indeed, farmed fish are fed more antibiotics per pound that any other animal raised for slaughter. (Check out page 26 to see how antibiotics in our food can make antibiotics less effective at treating diseases in humans.)

And finally, let's not forget sea lice. These little creeps, common in fish farms, attack the fish's organs, eventually eating them alive. These lice from farmed salmon are now spreading out to wild populations of fish in parts of the North Atlantic, meaning that soon, hiding under the sprig of parsley on your fresh fish, might be a spray of . . . well, you know.

# 22

# RAIN FORESTS
# ARE THE LUNGS
# OF THE PLANET

J oni Mitchell once sang that they paved paradise and put up a parking lot. It turns out she was almost right: They've paved paradise, but instead of putting up a parking lot, they're putting up feedlots.

Rain forests, which are home to more than half of the earth's animals and plants, once covered about 14 percent of the earth's land surface. Today, that percentage is down to 6.[37] Some scientists say that within fifty years, we will have eradicated almost all rain forests. In the Amazon rain forest alone, a soccer field–size tract of land is bulldozed every minute, chiefly to create room for livestock. The Amazon essentially acts as an enormous carbon vacuum that sucks up around 20 percent of the world's greenhouse gases, but over the past four decades, nearly one-fifth of the Amazon rain forest has been destroyed. All told, 80 to 90 percent of the deforestation is caused by cattle ranching.[38] (Remember that cows produce the methane equivalent of 3.1 gigatons of carbon dioxide per day.[39] Overall, livestock farming contributes roughly 18 percent of all human-caused greenhouse gas emissions worldwide.)

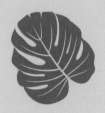

## DE(RAIN)FORESTATION:

Rain forests once covered about 14 percent of the earth's land surface. Today, that percentage is down to 6.

The cattle industry has ballooned since the 1970s, giving Brazil the largest commercial cattle herd in the world. Rather than help save the Amazon region, in 2019 the president of Brazil, Jair Bolsonaro, made it his business to encourage more ranching (as well as mining and logging) in the rain forest. Brazil's section of the Amazon lost more than 1,330 square miles[40] of forest during the first seven months of Bolsonaro's presidency—a more than 39 percent increase over the same period the previous year. Bolsonaro defended his actions, explaining that "Brazil is like a virgin that every pervert from the outside lusts for."

If we continue to hand our rain forests over to the cattle business, we will not only lose the heart and lungs of our planet, we will also lose a staggering number of animals and plants—especially fruits and vegetables that are critical to our well-being.

Eat plants. Save trees. Breathe better.

# WE'RE RUNNING
# OUT OF WATER

G et ready to feel thirsty. And slightly panicked. Check this out: Only about 2.5 percent of the water on our planet is fresh, and only 1 percent of that is readily available for human consumption. (The rest of it is locked up in icebergs and glaciers.) But where does a lot of that fresh water go? Not showers or iced tea or toilets. Rather, it goes to livestock.

> **One pound of meat takes about 1,800 gallons of water to produce.**

It's not that cows and sheep drink all the water. It's that the crops required to keep them fed use up a ton of water—to be specific, it takes nearly 150 gallons of water to produce 1 pound of corn and 220 gallons of water to produce 1 pound of soy. The average cow consumes some 750 pounds of feed each month until she's ready to be butchered, which is between two and three years. All told, that single cow will take in the equivalent of 183,000 gallons of water.[41]

Add to that all the water used for hydration, power-washing excrement from stalls, and cleaning the heavy machinery used during slaughter. Overall, one pound of meat takes about 1,800 gallons of water to produce.[42] That's the equivalent of doing forty loads of laundry or growing fifty-three pounds of potatoes. According to the American Meat Institute, the United States produces some 26 billion pounds of beef each year.[43] That comes out to 65 *trillion* gallons of water needed to produce America's beef.[44]

And dairy? Also terrible. Most dairy cows eat alfalfa, which is a water-intensive crop—one pound requires about 114 gallons of water. The average cow needs six pounds of alfalfa to produce one gallon of milk. If a dairy cow produces seven gallons of milk a day, that means 4,788 gallons of water. And again, that doesn't take into account any water the cow drinks.

Now think about how the average family of four uses 300 gallons of water a day for drinking, showers, cleaning, flushing, and so on. Add to that the water used to produce all the meat the average American eats, and that figure rises to over *ten thousand gallons* of water per year, per person.

A recent United Nations study estimates that by 2050, nearly half of the world's population will suffer from water scarcity.[45] So maybe it's time to consider redistributing those trillions of gallons of water used to maintain the livestock industry. Our lives depend on it.

# THE NUMBERS
# DON'T LIE

I t's time for pure data. Nothing touchy-feely. Noam Mohr, a physicist with degrees from Yale University and the University of Pennsylvania, has worked with the US Public Interest Research Group and EarthSave International on researching the specific impact of eating meat, dairy, and eggs on global warming. He has taken into consideration what animals are fed, in what manner they are raised and slaughtered, and how their carcasses and by-products are transported. He's gathered statistics on how the average American eats on a daily basis, and he's woven into consideration the effects of importing and exporting everything to do with livestock when it applies to the number of animals killed. Without further ado . . .

If every American went vegan for just one day, the United States would save[46]:

- 90 billion gallons of water, enough to supply all American homes for a week

- 2.8 million acres of land (which could be returned to its natural state of wilderness, such as forests and prairies)

- The fossil fuels equivalent to 78 million gallons of gas

If every American went vegan for just one day, the United States would prevent:

- Greenhouse gas emissions equivalent to 1.2 million tons of $CO_2$

- 4.75 million tons of animal excrement (a major source of water and air pollution), more than produced by the entire American population in four months

One American going vegan would save the United States:

- 180,000 gallons of water each year—that's 500 gallons each day

- 1,400 pounds of plant food otherwise fed to livestock each year—that's 4 pounds each day, which could feed the hungry and poor

- The fossil fuels equivalent of 87 gallons of gas each year

- More than 3 acres of land a year—that is, when you add up all the math, every extra day a person goes vegan each year theoretically saves another 375 square feet of wilderness

- Greenhouse gas emissions equivalent to 1.6 tons of $CO_2$ per year—that's 9 pounds each day

- More than 5 tons of animal excrement each year—that's 29 pounds each day

- $1/10$ of a pound of antibiotics each year—that's 128 mg per day, or like taking a typical dose every other day

Sit with the numbers awhile. Take out your calculator if it helps, and if you're interested in more global numbers, check out Faunalytics.org. Then bask in your power to effect change.

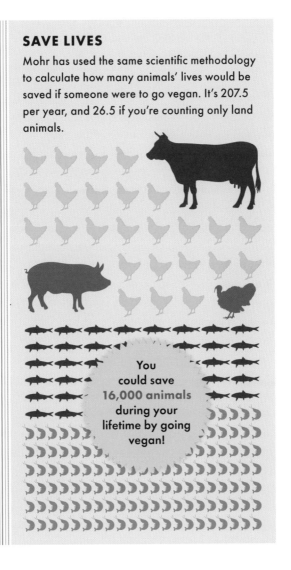

**SAVE LIVES**

Mohr has used the same scientific methodology to calculate how many animals' lives would be saved if someone were to go vegan. It's 207.5 per year, and 26.5 if you're counting only land animals.

You could save **16,000 animals** during your lifetime by going vegan!

# 2 5

# ANIMALS
# DESERVE
# BETTER

I n 2019, cats all over New York had cause for celebration: The state banned the cruel practice of declawing. That's great news for cats and for people who love cats (though maybe not so much for couches).

But what about the other animals who endure far worse than declawing? Sadly, New York's recent desire to prevent animal cruelty does not extend beyond pets. Without getting overly gross (which we could do very fast), here are just a few examples: Male pigs are routinely castrated in order to prevent them from giving off an odor known as "boar taint." This even happens to so-called "humanely raised" pigs, unless they're raised for breeding. And it happens without pain killers when the little piglets are only two weeks old. Ouch.

Bulls are also castrated, which makes the animals fatten up faster and, not surprisingly, makes them more compliant. We won't go into how it's done because you really don't want to know. Cattle are brutally dehorned—usually without painkillers—with searing-hot irons, caustic chemicals, blades, or even just handsaws. If the cow struggles too much, she is placed in a restraint. According to Dr. William Muir, a professor of animal sciences at Purdue University, dehorning is a "bloody . . . process that no one likes to do."[47] Yet people do it. Many millions of times a year.

Cattle continue to be branded, which is unfathomably painful and oddly anachronistic, as there are many more modern and pain-free ways to keep track of individual animals.

Because egg-laying hens are packed together in cages, they fight one another, as any terrified creature would. For this reason, their handlers routinely debeak them using a scalding hot knife when they are less than three weeks old, leaving them wounded, bleeding, and sometimes unable to eat again. Turkeys are similarly raised en masse on factory farms, packed together in tight, windowless spaces, their beaks and toes having been removed without anesthesia.

Little lambs, within weeks of being born, have their ears hole-punched and their tails chopped off; the males are castrated—(you guessed it) without anesthesia. In Australia, says a PETA report, ranchers simply carve "huge strips of flesh off the backs of lambs' legs and around their tails" to keep flies from laying eggs in the skin, as the hatched maggots can eat the sheep alive.[48]

All this is just the tip of the iceberg. What happens to animals being pushed through the slaughter line is truly horrific: They are typically dunked in scalding water (chickens), hung up by their legs (pigs), or sliced open (cows and pigs and chickens) sometimes while still alive. There's a reason we're not allowed into factory farms, and why slaughterhouses don't have windows.

# MEAT AND DAIRY
# ADDICTION IS REAL

Just as you can be addicted to cocaine or caffeine, you can also jones for meat and dairy. A 2015 study by researchers from the University of Michigan indicates that the more highly processed and fatty a food is, the more likely it is to cause addictive eating behavior.[49]

Cheese is addictive because of its casein content. Casein is a milk protein that breaks apart during digestion and releases a veritable army of opiates called casomorphins. According to the University of Illinois Extension Program, caseins comprise approximately 80 percent of the proteins in cow's milk.[50] And myriad studies have demonstrated that these casomorphins attach themselves to the very same brain receptors as heroin and cocaine.

According to Dr. Neal Barnard, founding president of the Physicians Committee for Responsible Medicine and the author of *The Cheese Trap*, it takes as many as three weeks to kick your craving for cheese.

Likewise, the blood in meat also contains chemicals that activate opioid receptors. According to one study by researchers in Edinburgh, Scotland, when meat-eaters were treated with a drug used to block opiate receptors, the volunteers subsequently chose to eat 10 percent less ham, 25 percent less salami, and 50 percent less tuna.[51]

## ARE YOU A MEATAHOLIC?

Curious to see if you're a meat or cheese addict? Many doctors use the Yale Food Addiction Scale to test for potential food addictions. The more you answer "yes," the more you might want to think about your relationship with meat and cheese.

- Do you continue to eat certain foods even when you are no longer hungry?

- Do you eat to the point of feeling physically ill?

- Do you find that when certain foods are not available, you'll go out of your way to obtain them?

- Do you constantly eat certain foods throughout the day?

- Do you have intense cravings?

- Are certain foods harder than others for you to stop eating?

- Do you ever choose to eat rather than spend time with friends and family?

- Do you ever avoid activities that you once enjoyed because you fear you might overeat at them?

- Has your overeating restricted your lifestyle?

- Have you ever avoided professional or social situations because you knew certain foods wouldn't be served there?

- Have you ever tried and failed to cut down or stop eating certain kinds of food?

- Does your behavior with respect to eating ever cause you significant distress?

**JUST THE FACTS:**

When scientists compared the five eating styles of 840 study participants, ranging from vegan to nonvegetarian, they discovered vegan bodies contained the most antioxidants.

# YOU CAN LIVE LONG
# AND PROSPER

A 2019 study published in *The Journal of Nutrition* followed 840 people who were divided into five eating styles: vegans, lacto-ovo vegetarians (eggs and dairy, but no fish or meat), pesco-vegetarians (also known as pescatarians—fish, but not meat), semi-vegetarians (meat eaten more than once a month, less than once a week), and nonvegetarians (sigh).[52] The study found that the bodies of vegans contained the most antioxidants, which, if you've been paying no attention to health trends over the last few decades, are substances—such as vitamins C and E, plant pigments like carotenoids, and minerals like selenium—that zap away free radicals, these ne'er-do-well molecules that harm our bodies' cellular structure. Surprisingly, vegans also had the most omega-3 fatty acids, a health-promoting fat that most people associate with consuming fatty fish, but which vegans obtain from walnuts, flaxseeds, and chia seeds.

All in all, unprocessed, plant-based foods tend to be healthier than animal-based ones because they are cholesterol-free (see page 130): they are lower in saturated fat; and they are higher in fiber, complex carbohydrates, and other essential nutrients. They are also an excellent source of protein, and brimming with vitamins, minerals, and phytonutrients.

As a result, vegans tend to have healthier microbiomes, lower blood pressure, lower incidence of diabetes, lower incidence of heart disease, and lower incidence of cancer. There's a reason why nutrition experts have written numerous best-selling books with titles like *Prevent and Reverse Heart Disease* (Dr. Caldwell Esselstyn), *How Not to Die* (Dr. Michael Greger), and *Dr. Neal Barnard's Program for Reversing Diabetes* (Dr. Neal Barnard).

More proof? A 2019 study published in *JAMA Internal Medicine* followed more than 70,000 Japanese men and women for an average of eighteen years.[53] After adjusting for various health and behavioral characteristics, the researchers found that, compared with the one-fifth of the group who ate the least plant protein (meaning they were getting the bulk of their protein from animal sources), the one-fifth who consumed the most had a 27 percent lower rate of cardiovascular death, a 28 percent lower rate of death from heart disease, and a 28 percent lower rate of stroke.

**Heart disease, cancer, and diabetes are extremely expensive.**

And the prosper part? Heart disease, cancer, and diabetes are not only extremely expensive to deal with, they also steal your energy and time—both of which could be better spent building a beautiful life.

# PLANT PROTEIN
# IS CLEAN PROTEIN

P rotein is crucial for building and repairing tissue and bones, producing essential enzymes and hormones, and countless other functions—we can't live without it—but not all protein is created equal. While plant protein is extremely healthy, animal protein is rife with problems. These include:

- High concentration of cholesterol and saturated fat (even fish and the white meat of chicken have a lot of cholesterol)

- Frequent contamination from *Salmonella*, *Campylobacter*, *E. coli*, *Listeria*, and so on[54]

- Drug and antibiotic residue (the crap they pump animals up with to make them put on weight before slaughter)[55]

- Hormones (more crap they pump animals up with to make them put on weight before slaughter)

- Extreme overuse and befouling of land and water associated with raising livestock

- Global warming gases generated by the livestock and meat industry

- A guilty conscience that comes from knowing what an animal went through before ending up on a dinner plate

Protein from plants, on the other hand, is *clean* protein, and:

- Has lots of fiber, which cleans you out (see page 21)

- Is 100 percent free of cholesterol and has very little, if any, saturated fat

- Has lots of antioxidants and phytonutrients

- Doesn't pollute our land and water, like livestock does

- Is not contaminated with pathogens (most contamination of plants comes from farmed animal waste or human carelessness, such as not washing hands; plants do not poop—see page 79)

- Is not responsible for even a fraction of the global warming gases associated with animal-based protein

- Makes no animals suffer, which leaves a clean conscience

Where do you get your protein if not from animals? The most concentrated sources are:

- Legumes (black beans, cannellini beans, pinto beans, lima beans, black-eyed peas)

- Nuts and nut butters

- Plant-based meat alternatives (hello, burgers!)

- Quinoa and amaranth

- Soy (tofu, tempeh, edamame)

- Seeds (hemp, flax, chia, pumpkin, sunflower, sesame)

- Hummus (chickpeas and tahini)

- Vegan protein powder (made from peas, rice, soy, or hemp)

- Whole grains (oats, wild rice, spelt, millet, wheat, barley)

- High-protein bean pasta

There's protein in everything; it's just a matter of eating enough calories from whole plant-based foods. The official daily recommendation is 0.36 grams of protein for every pound you weigh.[56] So, if you weigh 150 pounds, shoot for 54 grams of protein per day. If you're pregnant, lactating, or are an athlete in training, the goal is closer to 67.5 grams of protein per day, but be sure to check with your doctor.

Now, you might have heard the old wives' tale that plant-based protein isn't "complete." Wrong! Plant protein is completely complete. Protein is made up from a variety of amino acids, and amino acids are in both animal and plant foods. Animal proteins and certain plant proteins are called "complete proteins" because they contain some amount of all the essential amino acids. But that *doesn't mean they're better*, because the body naturally combines amino acids from different food sources into proteins. So it takes some amino acids from the oats or rice you're eating and pairs them with those from the lentils from your soup, and voila, you have your complete protein! And you don't have to eat grains and beans together at the same meal to get the complete package; as long as you're eating a diverse diet over the course of a few days, you're getting everything you need and then some.

The takeaway: The cleanest possible delivery of protein is through plant-based sources; it's cholesterol-free, hormone-free, antibiotic-free, and cruelty-free. You'll get everything you need, nothing you don't, and a whole lot of good vibes. #AnimalFreeDiet.

# YOUR GUT WILL
# THANK YOU

If you're looking for something to worry about, think about your gut. Those thirty feet of internal organs, today known as your gut microbiome, are a key factor in your overall health.

What actually is a gut? And what is its microbiome (aka the trillions of microbes living in your body)?

Anatomically speaking, your "gut" doesn't refer to a specific organ, but rather a number of them—your stomach, gallbladder, small intestine, large intestine, pancreas, and liver—that collectively make up the digestive system. However, when most people say "gut," they mean the colon, that is, your large intestine, which gets its name because it's about five feet long. Inside it reside trillions (yes, trillions) of bacteria, viruses, fungi, and more. Indeed, you have more bacteria living in your body (forty trillion) that you have cells (thirty trillion). And the bacteria weigh about three pounds, or nearly as much as your brain. You are, in essence, a walking, talking sack of bacteria.

These bacteria (and there are as many as a thousand different species swimming around you this very minute) have all kinds of tasks. They help you digest fiber (see page 21), they help control your immune system, they affect your heart, they can lower the risk of diabetes, they even help control your central nervous system.

But they don't do only good things. And when bad bacteria take over from good bacteria in your gut microbiome, they might raise your risk of anything from an upset stomach to irritable bowel syndrome to weight gain to colorectal cancer.[57]

Having a healthy microbiome is essential to good health. There's no surprise that one of the best ways to get that microbiome in good shape is to eat a diet low in saturated fat, salt, and added sugars, and high in legumes, vegetables, seeds, fruits, and whole grains.

Hmmm. That's a vegan diet.

According to a 2019 study published in *Frontiers in Nutrition*, "Current research indicates that . . . a plant-based diet may be an effective way to promote a diverse ecosystem of beneficial microbes that support overall health."[58]

According to the Physicians Committee for Responsible Medicine, the best ways to increase the good bacteria in your gut are to:

- Avoid animal products.

- Avoid fried foods.

- Avoid unnecessary antibiotics, which can destroy your microbiome. Unless you absolutely need antibiotics, don't take them.

- Fill up on fiber.

- Eat prebiotic-rich foods (ones that feed healthy bacteria), such as onions, garlic, asparagus, and whole wheat, as well as probiotic foods, including sauerkraut, miso, tempeh, and kimchi.

- Practice a healthy lifestyle; don't just think about your diet, but also make sure you get enough sleep and exercise.

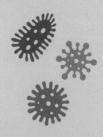

**SPOILER ALERT:**

**One of the best ways to get your microbiome in good shape is to eat a vegan diet.**

# MARTINIS.

## COFFEE. FUN.

L ife is meant to be enjoyed; no one is interested in subsisting on boring bowls of lettuce and steamed broccoli. Yeesh, no thanks. Nor are we all interested in meditating for long stretches of the day or sermonizing about what's wrong with the world or wagging our fingers at what must be changed right now! (Not that there's anything wrong with that.) People often used to think that vegans lived like righteous monks. That just ain't so.

We're as fun-loving as everyone else, and eating good food is a big part of feeling alive and connected. Are we interested in being healthy? Sure, but not so much that we can't partake in life's pleasures from time to time. Kathy loves vodka martinis and Gene likes a little cannabis—both are vegan. Vegan pizza and Beyond Burgers may not be considered health foods, but they're a helluva lot better than eating the trans fat– and cholesterol-filled animal proteins, or dealing with the environmental destruction and cruelty associated with eating meat and cheese. You can enjoy your cup of joe in the morning; it's just a matter of subbing out the cow's milk for soy creamer or oat milk. You get the same buzz, but without the lactose hangover.

This way of living brings joy, and it feels good. Your body feels good because you have more energy to be present in life and appreciative of all it has to offer. Your mind feels good because your brain is sharp and you've figured out how to become part of the solution instead of the problem. You feel more plugged in to your community because you know you are helping lift it to a better place. You feel sexy, and your improved circulation makes all the parts work correctly. You feel confident because people notice something different about you, and they want to know your secret.

## YOU WON'T MISS A THING

From oat milk to cashew cheese to coconut milk yogurt, plants have you pretty much covered with these meat and dairy substitutes.

- Oat *milk*
- Cashew *cheese*
- Coconut *yogurt*
- Plant-based *burgers*
- Vegan *sausages*
- Cheesy *pizza*
- Vegetable *broth*
- Oat-milk *ice cream*
- Soy *ricotta*
- Pea *protein powder*
- Mung bean *eggs*
- Tempeh *bacon*
- Jackfruit *brisket*
- Eggless *mayo*
- Aquafaba *meringue*
- Legume-based *seafood*
- Seitan *roast*
- Mock meat *cold cuts*
- Tofu *cheesecake*
- Vegan *butter*
- Soy *cream cheese*
- Mushroom *steak*
- Nooch *parmesan cheese*

So, carry on, relax, and enjoy. Most of what you have in your daily mix is already vegan—all the fixings on the sandwich or burger, the fries on the side, the stuff in your smoothie; you just need to switch out that animal dreck for a cleaner protein. If you eat a muffin with some egg in it, don't worry; just look for a better version on the next go-around. You don't need to torture waiters or be the creep at the dinner party; think of this journey like a sport you're learning. Get better at it all the time and have fun on the way!

None of us should be forced to white-knuckle our way through life, saying no to foods that make us feel content. There are plenty of things that are fun and (or can be) vegan: burgers and fries, Oreo cookies, sex, movies, popcorn, dancing, protein smoothies, cannabis, ice pops at the beach, hanging out with your friends and pets, sandwiches, traveling to new places, daydreaming, cocktails with friends. All you need to do is to keep making progress, and don't worry about perfection. You don't have to live on a higher plane of existence and be holier-than-thou toward everyone else. You don't have to go to vegan-only restaurants and have vegan-only friends. And you certainly don't have to give up all your vices!

# THE WORLD
# IS BECOMING
# OVERRUN WITH
# ANIMAL POOP

Benjamin Franklin once said that "nothing can be said to be certain, except death and taxes." He could have added another certainty: poop. Animal poop. It's everywhere, and it's not going away. In the United States alone, livestock produce approximately 396 million tons of excrement every year.[59]

Think that's a load of crap? The farmed animals who occupy some 45 percent of the planet's surface are doing far more than occupying it. They are crapping all over it. Hills of it, mountains of it, draining into our land and water supplies. The average beef cow eats around 90 pounds of food a day, and poops 15 times a day. That's about 65 pounds of poop a day, or close to 12 tons of poop a year. A lactating cow poops nearly 150 pounds worth every day. Every day. That's 27 tons a year. And that's just the cows. Think of the pigs, the sheep, and the chickens. All these animals are pooping every day, and there are fewer and fewer places to put or treat it.

Unlike human poop, which goes through sewage processing plants, this poop is generally stored in waste lagoons or sprayed over fields as fertilizer. The runoff from all this poop is one of the primary causes of pollution in rivers and lakes. The toxic runoff carries nitrates, phosphorous, bacteria, and viruses that contaminate nearby groundwater, which can kill fish and harm people. In fact, large-scale industrial factory farms are one of the leading causes of drinking water contamination nation-wide. All because of poop.

**FECAL FACT:** Poop pollutes the air as much as the water. Waste emits scores of dangerous gases, including hydrogen sulfide, which can cause eye, nose, and throat irritation, and ammonia, which at high levels is very toxic. The air around factory farms also becomes contaminated with suspended dust particles, which have been linked to asthma, bronchitis, and other serious health concerns.

One recent North Carolina study of 58,000 children found a 23 percent higher prevalence of asthma symptoms among students who attended schools located near factory farms.[60] Other analyses have discovered links between waste and neurological and respiratory problems.

# THERE IS NO SUCH THING AS HUMANE SLAUGHTER

When you see a "humanely raised" label on a package of meat—which likely came from a factory farm, not some bucolic family farm of yesteryear—it means absolutely nothing other than that the brand had a good marketing team. Such a label does not mean the animals were happy; it only means that the ad agency knows what customers need to see in order to feel good about what they're drinking or eating.

Take the phrase "free range": The label can simply mean that there's a tiny little door on a faraway wall in a massive shed through which a chicken could theoretically wander—that is, if she could navigate through tens of thousands of other chickens first. Moreover, consider that by the time broiler chickens are forty days old and plump for slaughter, many cannot walk because they have been genetically bred to put on crippling amounts of fat, which fetches more money per pound.

And "grass fed." Yes, it's nice that the animals have a healthier diet of grass. They get some sunshine while they are fattened up; they can move their legs unlike their factory-farmed counterparts. Frankly, though, that might even be worse because the animal got a taste of freedom before she was

**THE REALITY:**

The vast majority (around 97 percent) of animals killed for food are factory farmed; only a tiny percentage are from genuine small family farms.

loaded up on a truck and carted off to the same dismal slaughterhouses that every other food animal is killed in. Interestingly, recent studies suggest that grass-fed cows actually produce *more* of the potent greenhouse gas methane compared with their counterparts raised on feedlots.[61] So, by being marginally less cruel to cows, we are being even more cruel to the environment. When it comes to eating meat, there truly is no good way.

Now imagine you're a 43-day-old chicken at the slaughterhouse, where you're aggressively hustled into long, confusing, terrifying lines. The workers seem mad at you; they're hurting you, rushing you, and you fight to turn around but you can't, and then . . . you smell blood and flesh and crap. You hear god-awful sounds from other animals. What's happening, what's happening . . . and then a stun in your head. But you're still alive; they missed. And swoop, you're hung up by your feet and something horrible is about to happen.

You get the drift. When people say, "Hey, the animal had a good life and then one bad day," well, it's not just a bad day. It's a horrific day in the slaughterhouse, the same slaughterhouse where every factory-farmed or "humanely raised" animal ends up, where animals fight for their lives as they progress through the lines in terror.

On an economic note, the vast majority (around 97 percent) of animals killed for food are factory farmed; only a tiny percentage are from genuine small family farms. That tiny percentage of meat is very expensive and out of reach for most people, whether they're eating at home or at a high-end restaurant.

# 33

# WORKING AT A SLAUGHTERHOUSE IS HELL

Job opportunity posting for a slaughterhouse worker. Tasks, expectations, and responsibilities include the following:

- Remove bones and cut meat into standard cuts in preparation for marketing.

- Sever jugular veins to drain blood and facilitate slaughtering.

- Tend to assembly lines, performing a few of the many cuts needed to process a carcass.

- Shackle hind legs of animals to raise them for slaughtering or skinning.

- Slit open, eviscerate, and trim carcasses of slaughtered animals.

- Stun animals prior to slaughtering.

- Shave or singe and defeather carcasses; wash them in preparation for further processing or packaging.

- Saw, split, or scribe carcasses into smaller portions to facilitate handling.

- Skin sections of animals or whole animals.

- Trim head meat and sever or remove parts of animals' heads or skulls.

- Grind meat into hamburger and into trimmings used to prepare sausages, luncheon meats, and other meat products.

- Trim, clean, or cure animal hides.

- Wrap dressed carcasses or meat cuts.

Being a slaughterhouse worker is as dehumanizing as you might imagine. Still, many people simply need a paying job and will accept whatever they must to support their families. But this is a cruel blow. Workers in slaughterhouses suffer terrible working conditions: It's astoundingly loud (the combination of animals in extreme distress and heavy machinery), the floors are thick with blood, and it's very physical and dangerous work. It's not surprising that workers endure a high rate of alcoholism and PTSD. And even with the need to make money, slaughterhouse workers don't tend to last long on the job. In her seminal exposé, *Slaughterhouse*, Gail Eisnitz writes that "according to the United Food and Commercial Workers International Union, which represents thousands of slaughterhouse employees, the worker turnover rate in high-speed plants approached 100 percent per year."

As the Food Empowerment Project points out, "In their endless goal of higher volume and greater efficiency, these corporations knowingly jeopardize workers' safety every day."[62] To save money, slaughterhouses often knowingly hire undocumented workers living in some of the poorest communities in the country. As much as 38 percent of all slaughterhouse and processing-plant workers were born outside of the United States, and many of them are paid below the minimum wage. If they complain, they are fired and replaced—or worse, threatened with deportation.

And you might recall that American slaughterhouses became hotspots for the spread of COVID-19 infections due to frigid temperatures inside the meatpacking plants, a general lack of personal protective equipment for the employees who stand shoulder to shoulder as they work, and long hours of grueling labor—and that's on top of the regular injuries and PTSD from working in these places.

# LAUGHING GAS
# IS NOT SO FUNNY

Nitrous oxide, commonly known as laughing gas, is great in small doses if you're waiting for your dentist to remove your tooth. However, nitrous oxide is about three hundred times more potent a greenhouse gas than carbon dioxide. Best we prevent this dangerous gas from leaking into the atmosphere, right? According to the United Nations, the meat, egg, and dairy industries account for 65 percent of worldwide nitrous oxide emissions. That's because livestock feed typically requires large applications of nitrogen-based fertilizer, which turns into nitrous oxide in the ground. It's also released into the air during the storage and treatment of livestock manure. Not a laughing matter.

# IT'S GOOD FOR
# GROWING KIDS!

But what about the kiddos, you may ask? Is an animal-free diet okay for them, too? Sure is.

Kids today are in the worst physical shape of any generation in history. One in three is overweight. One in five teenagers has high cholesterol. According to the Centers for Disease Control, one in three kids born in 2000 will get a diagnosis of diabetes at some point in their life. But a kid who chooses to eat whole plant foods rather than animals has a near certainty of avoiding high cholesterol, high blood pressure, obesity, and other symptoms of heart disease.

And in case you're worried about a kid being as tall or strong as the others their age, researchers studied a group of 1,765 children and adolescents in Southern California, and vegetarians were, on average, about an inch taller than their meat-eating friends.

But take it from Dr. Neal Barnard, whom we heard from on page 64. He explains that "vegan children have better nutrition than other kids. This is in part because they are skipping the cholesterol and animal fat, and in part because as they search for new foods to eat (to replace the meat), they often discover and start eating healthy foods. While all kids are supposed to eat their veggies, according to the ADA, vegan and vegetarian kids actually do!"[63]

And according to Dr. Michael Greger, author of *How Not to Die*: "Heart disease starts in childhood. By age 10, nearly all kids have fatty streaks in their arteries. This is the first sign of atherosclerosis, the leading cause of death in the United States."[64] Dr. Greger points out that studies show that heart disease can even begin in the womb, depending on the diet and cholesterol level of the mother.

So, in other words, it's never too early to go vegan. Here are two simple rules that ensure good nutrition:

1    Each day, have foods from the four healthful food groups: whole grains, legumes (beans, peas, and lentils), vegetables, and fruits.

2    Include a reliable source of vitamin $B_{12}$, such as a supplement or fortified foods (cereals and plant-based milks, for example).

Dr. Barnard goes on to say, "If you are interested in trying soy-based meat substitutes, they may have health benefits. Girls who consume soy milk, tofu, or similar products on a daily basis during adolescence have significantly less risk of breast cancer in adulthood, compared to people who avoid soy. That said, soy products are not essential. There is plenty of good nutrition in the other beans, as well as in the broad range of vegetables, fruits, and grains."

Yeah, but how do you get a kid to eat this way, you may ask? Start gradually: Begin with

## WHAT ALL KIDS NEED

Here's a closer look at a few key nutrients that are critical for growing kids.

**PROTEIN:** There is ample protein in grains, vegetables, beans, and bean products (including tofu and soy milk). If your child consumes a normal variety of these foods over the course of a day, she will receive all the protein she needs. (Subtext: A child cannot thrive on pasta alone.)

**CALCIUM:** Green leafy vegetables and legumes, or "greens and beans," are rich in calcium. This is particularly true for broccoli, collards, kale, bok choy, and Brussels sprouts. You'll also find plenty of calcium in fortified foods, such as fortified orange juice and most soy milks. And don't fight over vegetables your child doesn't like. Just serve the ones that do go over well. Tastes broaden as the years go by.

**IRON:** Greens and beans come to our rescue again. They are rich in iron, and vitamin C–rich foods, such as citrus fruits, tend to enhance the absorption of iron consumed in the same meal.

**VITAMIN B$_{12}$:** Many fortified breakfast cereals and plant milks contain vitamin B$_{12}$, which is essential for healthy blood and healthy nerves.

Meatless Mondays as a family, and then progress to eating less and less meat while you're all getting more comfortable with the fresher fare. What kid doesn't like a taco or burrito? Just fill them with beans and rice instead of meat, and top with guacamole and shredded lettuce. You can use veggie meatballs in pasta, or plant-based chicken fingers heated in the toaster oven. Pizza is easy, too, because there are loads of vegan cheeses on the market. And cue up the smoothies; they taste like dessert to a kid, but you can load them with frozen veggies and fruits and they'll never know they're getting healthy stuff. (Frozen blueberries and frozen broccoli are the best way to get your children into eating veggies, because the berries make a smoothie wonderfully purple and the kids won't even taste the broccoli.)

**It's never too early to go vegan.**

Be really happy about a kid who wants to go vegan. Odds are they will grow up taller and healthier than their meat-eating counterparts. More importantly, they'll grow up to be kind and mindful global citizens.

# 3 6

# YOU WANT TO LIVE LONGER THAN A CAVEMAN

You've probably heard of the paleo diet, also known as the caveman diet. The theory goes that humans should be eating what they supposedly did two million years ago. That means copious amounts of meat, fish, fruits, vegetables, nuts, and seeds. We're on board with those last four items, but the first two, unfortunately, destroy all those good vibes.

The paleo diet sounded revolutionary when it gained a cult following about a decade ago, but it's actually been around for years. Take the Atkins diet, which demonizes carbs while encouraging protein-rich meat and eggs. Sound familiar? Both diets shun nearly all whole grains and beans. And with both, you generally can't even have your favorite legumes, including peanuts, beans, lentils, and tofu.

What does the science have to say about eating this way? In 2018, the European Society of Cardiology released the results of its landmark study comprising nearly twenty-five thousand people over more than a decade: "We found that people who consumed a low-carbohydrate diet were at greater risk of premature death. Risks were also increased for individual causes of death

## LET'S PUT IT THIS WAY:

The average life span of
a caveman during the
Paleolithic era was about
thirty to thirty-five years.

including coronary heart disease, stroke, and cancer. These diets should be avoided."[65] According to the study, when compared with people with the highest intake of carbs, those with the lowest intake had a "32% higher risk of all-cause death over an average 6.4-year follow-up. In addition, risks of death from coronary heart disease, cerebrovascular disease, and cancer were increased by 51%, 50%, and 35%, respectively."

A study out of the University of Melbourne found that just eight weeks on the paleo diet can lead to high blood pressure, bone problems, high blood sugar, and diabetes.[66] Meanwhile, a study published in the *European Journal of Clinical Nutrition* concluded that the diet increases levels of TMAO, a metabolite associated with heart disease.[67] It gets worse: Another study found that after ten weeks on the paleo diet, subjects' LDL—the "bad" cholesterol—jumped by over 12 percent, while total cholesterol ballooned by more than 6 percent.[68] As we know, elevated cholesterol levels are directly tied to an increased risk of congestive heart failure and a host of other chronic diseases.

If that's what fewer than three months of eating meat, dairy, and eggs can do to your body, imagine what an entire lifetime could do. Let's put it this way: The average life span of a caveman during the Paleolithic era was about thirty to thirty-five years. So, if you want to truly live and die like a caveman, perhaps this diet is for you. But if you want to live a long and healthy life in the twenty-first century, maybe you should stick to plants.

# YOU CAN UP
# YOUR GAME

Once upon a time, athletes wanting a performance boost would score some anabolic steroids, testosterone, HGH, or any number of other illicit drugs. They'd then probably have performed better and, oh, gotten busted, too. Just ask Lance Armstrong, Mark McGwire, or Barry Bonds. If only there were some safe, legal option, one that could help anyone trying to make some performance gains.

You're in luck. There's a vegan product that not only improves your marathon splits, but also reduces your blood pressure, among many other health benefits. It's legal, cheap, and you can find it in the produce aisle at your local supermarket. We're talking beets!

Okay, so beets don't sound like the most exciting food in the world. They're usually covered in dirt and look kind of lumpy. But these unassuming taproots are extremely potent. Take it from the title of this study: "Whole beetroot consumption acutely improves running performance." Published in the *Journal of the Academy of Nutrition and Dietetics*, scientists offered male and female athletes about a cup and a half of baked beets and had them run a 5K.[69] Guess what? The beet group pulled ahead of the control group, who were not given beets, during the final mile. All told, the beet dopers ran 5 percent faster while not working any harder—an enormous boost that even Nike and Adidas can't beat with their space-age soles and multimillion-dollar research budgets. Other studies have found that beet juice can help free divers hold their breath for an extra 30 seconds due to improved oxygen efficiency.

If only Lance had known about beets, he might still be considered an American icon. Just after he was busted, a 2012 study had twelve trained cyclists consume 140 mL of beet juice daily in the six days leading up to the trial. Sure enough, their average power output increased from 288 watts to 294 watts. That may not seem like a huge amount, but cyclists spend thousands of dollars on ultralight gear to see a 2 percent performance gain, which can be the difference between first place and fiftieth in a long race. Team Ineos, one of the most successful cycling teams today, spends millions of dollars finding ways to eke out marginal gains of just 0.5 percent, and beet juice is high on their list of prerace rituals.

**Natural nitrates found in beets increase your body's ability to extract energy from oxygen.**

It turns out that the natural nitrates found in beets not only cause your arteries to dilate, which helps deliver more oxygen-rich blood to your muscles, but they also increase your body's ability to extract energy from oxygen. But you don't have to be a finely tuned athlete to reap the benefits: If you are at risk of heart disease, beets have been shown in many studies to help reduce blood pressure. High blood pressure, or hypertension, means your heart muscle thickens, requiring more force to pump blood. This can damage your arteries and make them stiffer, raising your risk of heart failure. Beets—along with other vegetables including cabbage, celery, chervil, spinach, cress, dill, and lettuce—contain nitric oxide, which helps your blood vessels relax, improving blood flow and reducing blood pressure. In a 2016 study, individuals suffering from hypertension who began drinking beet juice saw their systolic blood pressure drop 14 points on average after just a few weeks.[70] Among heart disease patients, that can be the difference between life and death.

# CREAMY
# DOESN'T HAVE
# TO MEAN DAIRY

D o not worry: You *do not* have to give up cream to go vegan! Repeat: You will not miss out on creaminess by giving up animal stuff! You can have Alfredo sauce on your pasta, rich and velvety soups, desserts drizzled with decadent cream sauce, and everything else your little taste buds desire.

Say hello to the mighty cashew.

Cashews are awesome because they don't have a strong, nutty taste. And they have a good bit of fat in them, which makes them rich. When blended with water, they make a decadent cream that rivals anything that comes from cows.

How to make it: Take a handful of raw, unsalted cashews and soak them in water overnight, which softens them up and makes them easier to digest. If you forget to do it overnight, just soak them in hot water for as long as you have time for.

Drain the soaking water and toss the cashews into a high-powered blender with some water— how much depends on how thick you want your cream to be. A good basic ratio to start with is 1:2 (1 cup cashews to 2 cups fresh water), and then you can make as much or little as you like, as thin or thick as you prefer. Blend on high speed, while occasionally stopping to scrape down the sides of your blender.

You can add a date or sugar to sweeten the cream, and use it as a pudding or dessert sauce on top of cake or a brownie. You can add nutritional yeast, a little bit of lemon, and salt to make a cheesy sauce for veggies or pasta. Or you can add vegetable broth and steamed vegetables into the blender for a cream of asparagus (or mushroom or broccoli) soup. Get creative with whatever flavors you want to mix into it, such as vanilla, maple syrup, garlic, black or red pepper, or whatever spice you have a hankering for.

Then just add a dollop of it to whatever you think needs a creamy touch. We like the savory version of it drizzled over roasted vegetables as a snack or side dish; we love it on top of mashed potatoes and chickpea cakes; and we love it atop berry crumble for dessert. One of our favorite treats is pasta with vegan sausage and cashew cream sauce because it's flat-out decadent and there's not a meat-eater in the world who wouldn't flip over that meal. You don't even need a recipe for it; just sauté the sausages in the cream with garlic and salt, and voila!

Cashew cream lasts for about a week in the fridge, and you can freeze it, too. (Just take it out of the freezer and put it in the fridge overnight to thaw.) Thank you to our friend and genius vegan chef, Tal Ronnen, for introducing this heavenly knowledge into the zeitgeist.

# 39

# FOODBORNE ILLNESS IS KILLING US

*almonella. E. coli* O157:H7. *Listeria monocytogenes (Lm). Campylobacter.* Not exactly household names, but they are household presences. These bacteria and viruses are the top four causes of foodborne illness, a problem that sickens 48 million Americans each year, hospitalizes 128,000, and kills 3,000, according to the Centers for Disease Control.

Where do they come from? Foods are one source, but some foods are more responsible than others. According to a recent CDC report, animal foods collectively resulted in more illness than plant foods, with eggs linked to the highest number of *Salmonella* cases, beef to the most *E. coli* O157:H7, raw milk and soft cheeses to the most *Listeria*, and dairy to the most *Campylobacter.* Also, certain fatal diseases are found *only* in animal foods. These include brain-destroying Creutzfeldt-Jakob (or "Mad Cow") disease, caused by proteins called prions in sick beef cattle, and vibriosis, a nasty illness caused by the *Vibrio* bacteria found in shellfish, especially oysters.

That's why preparing meat, poultry, and seafood requires many careful steps to protect yourself and your family from pathogens. You know the drill: Don't let the raw flesh touch any countertops, utensils, or dishes, or you'll have to wipe them down with antimicrobial spray or run them through a hot dishwasher. Cook the food to a minimum internal temperature to kill all those germs. But don't char it *too* much, because overcooked meat produces cancer-causing compounds. Same with eggs and milk products: Don't eat unpasteurized dairy, because disease-causing microbes thrive there.

In other words, cook animal protein too little and risk foodborne illness. Cook it too much and risk cancer.

But with veggies and fruits? For the most part, you can simply wash the skins and eat them. Or, as with bananas or avocados, simply remove the skin before eating! No surprise, then, that the go-to website on this subject, StopFoodborneIllness.org, makes it clear that "a vegan diet does reduce risk of foodborne illness related to meals made with meats/eggs/dairy."

However, vegans should still pay attention to food safety, since produce can become

**FRUSTRATING FACT:** Lettuce has taken a lot of heat for recent E. coli outbreaks, but E. coli bacteria live in the intestines ("coli" comes from "colon") of animals. When plants become contaminated, it's because they came into contact with infected animal waste that was used to fertilize crops or that leaked into waterways. Either that, or some human didn't wash their hands before making a salad.

contaminated. Here are some simple tips adapted from the Stop Foodborne Illness site:

- Select unbruised fresh fruits and vegetables, which have a lesser chance of being contaminated.

- Properly clean produce. For tips, check out the opposite page, which is based on a fruit and veggie safety poster at CDC.gov/foodsafety.

- Store your produce properly to help it stay fresh longer.

- Prevent spoilage and bacterial growth by refrigerating or freezing cut-up produce and salads within a couple of hours (one hour if it's more than 90 degrees out).

# FRUIT & VEGETABLE SAFETY

These are steps that can help keep you healthy—and your fruits and vegetables safer to eat—from the store to your table.

## At the Store

- Select produce that is free of bruises or damaged spots, unless you plan to cook them.
- Choose precut and packaged fruits and vegetables that are refrigerated or kept on ice.
- Keep fruits and vegetables separate from raw meat, poultry, and seafood in your shopping cart and grocery bags.
- Get fruits and vegetables home and in the fridge in two hours or less.

## At Home

**WASH**

- Wash your hands before and after preparing produce.
- Wash or scrub all fruits and vegetables under running water before eating, cutting, or cooking.
- Fruits and vegetables labeled "prewashed" do not need to be washed again at home.

**KEEP COLD**

- Refrigerate cut, peeled, or cooked fruits and vegetables as soon as possible, or within two hours.
- Make sure the refrigerator temperature stays at 40°F or below.

**SEPARATE**

- Store produce away from, and not next to or below, raw meat, poultry, and seafood.
- Wash cutting boards, countertops, and utensils with hot, soapy water before and after preparing food.

*Source: CDC*

# 40

# PRO BODYBUILDERS CHOOSE VEGAN

A lot of people will try to convince you that if you're going to go vegan, you'll end up underweight with no muscle tone, sagging skin, and flabby limbs. Tell that to vegan Patrik Baboumian—who also happens to be one of the world's strongest men.

An Iranian who currently lives in Germany, Patrik started off his career by winning the German Junior Bodybuilding title in 1999. He then went on to hold several world log lift records, and eventually became the European Powerlifting Champion, not to mention the German Open Overall Champion, German Lightweight *and* Heavyweight Champion in Strongman, and the European Champion in Raw Powerlifting, among other competition records. And, in 2011, Patrik won Germany's Strongest Man contest.

Here's what Patrik said several years ago at the Toronto Veg fest: "This is a message to all those out there who think that you need animal products to be fit and strong. Almost two years after becoming vegan I am stronger than ever before and I am still improving day by day. Don't listen to those self-proclaimed nutrition gurus and the supplement industry trying to tell you that you need meat, eggs, and dairy to get enough protein. There are plenty of plant-based protein sources, and your body is going to thank you for [not] feeding it with dead food. Go vegan and feel the power!"[71]

By the way, according to Barbend.com, in the average day, Patrik eats (plant-based) food containing 5,320 calories, 410 grams of protein, 470 grams of carbs, and 200 grams of fat.

Other vegan bodybuilders include Nick Squires, a California-based powerlifter who has won numerous events; Anastasia Zinchenko, a British powerlifter with several regional UK titles; Glenda Presutti, an elite Australian powerlifter in her sixties who's been vegan since 2016; Nigel Morton, a Canadian lifter who was raised vegetarian and is now vegan; Bill McCarthy, an American powerlifter who has finished six times in the top five at the US Nationals—and many others.

> **"Your body is going to thank you for [not] feeding it with dead food."**

# PIGS ARE SMARTER
# THAN A THREE-YEAR-
# OLD CHILD

Babe. Wilbur. Pig Wig. Arnold Ziffel. The Oinker Sisters. Miss Piggy. Porky Pig.

Throughout books, movies, cartoons, and television, pigs have been stars. And they are stars in real life as well. Studies have shown them to be either the third or fourth most intelligent animal in the world, following, perhaps, chimps, dolphins, and elephants. (Humans aren't smart enough to know for sure.)

Like humans, pigs are very social animals; they can learn skills from one another, and they can complete tasks as a team. They never stop learning. A researcher at the University of Illinois found that pigs can even figure out how to control the thermostat of their barn. Anyone who has spent time with pigs will also attest to their wide range of personalities, as different as Wilbur is from Babe. Some are smarter, some are funnier, some are shyer; they are as distinct from each other as humans are. Also, like humans, they can empathize with each other.[72]

Pigs also like to talk. A lot. They are constantly chatting with each other, with at least twenty different oinks, grunts, snorts, and squeaks that all have meanings that other pigs understand. They tell each other, or you, how they feel, whom they like, and when they're hungry. It may turn out, after further study, that they have many dozens more utterances only they understand.

Countless stories detail how pigs have accomplished remarkable feats. They've saved humans, fellow pigs, and other animals from drowning, fires, and other dangers. One pig whose human friend was having a heart attack flagged down a car to get her help. Pigs display distress when they see animals, or humans, suffering. They learn to forgive as well: Pigs who have been rescued from horribly abusive situations can learn to love their new human companions, despite all that they have suffered in the past.

They are also much cleaner than we tend to give them credit for. Unlike other farm animals, pigs create separate sleeping and latrine areas. They roll around in mud, true, but that's because they have no sweat glands, and the mud cools them off. If you were to introduce them to an air-conditioned room, they'd forgo the mud. And, of course, they're adorably adorable. Go on Instagram and you can find scores of sweet playful pigs with photogenic personalities—and millions of followers. You can see them playing with people, or surfing the waves in Hawaii, or carrying kittens on their backs. The cuteness: It never stops.

**Only 3 percent of pigs ever see the outdoors.**

Now, given all this, why do we treat pigs the way we do? No one has a good answer. And yet, pregnant sows spend their lives in barren metal cages too small to let them turn around. Piglets are routinely castrated without painkillers. Sick piglets are slammed headfirst into concrete floors. We horribly mutilate their bodies. Only 3 percent of pigs ever see the outdoors. The list of terrible things we do to these animals is long and scary.

Why not head to a farm sanctuary and adopt a pig who needs your help? It'll make you feel a lot better than eating a ham sandwich ever could.

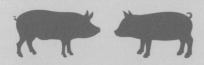

**PIG PATTER:**

**Pigs are constantly chatting with each other, with at least twenty different oinks, grunts, snorts, and squeaks that all have meanings that other pigs understand.**

# CHICKENS LIKE
# TO BE CUDDLED

Many people say, "I don't eat meat—just chicken." Say what?

Eating chicken is eating meat. It is the body of a dead animal. That's that.

But then they might say, "Well, chickens don't matter. They're not sentient beings. They can't feel pain."

Actually, they can. Just as scientists have been uncovering how remarkable pigs are, they've found chickens are pretty cool, too. Studies performed at the University of Padua, Italy, have shown that chickens can count; they can solve basic arithmetic problems, just like any school child. According to a study from the UK's University of Bristol, they show remarkable empathy toward each other.[73] They are very social animals and fully understand where they stand in their literal pecking order. And according to a study published in *Animal Cognition* in 2017, they can also "reason by deduction—an ability that humans develop by the age of seven." For example, newly hatched chicks presented with two sets of objects of varying amounts hidden behind two screens were able to perform simple mental arithmetic and determine which screen hid the larger amount.[74]

According to that same 2017 study, "Chicken communication is also quite complex, and consists of a large repertoire of different visual displays and at least 24 distinct vocalizations. The birds possess the complex ability of referential communication, which involves signals such as calls, displays and whistles to convey information. They may use this to sound the alarm when there is danger, for instance. This ability requires some level of self-awareness and being able to take the perspective of another animal, and is also possessed by highly intelligent and social species, including primates."

Like pigs and humans, chickens have very distinct personalities—some are fun-loving, some are arrogant, some are weird. By the way, you, human that you are, may think all chickens look alike, but not so to chickens; they can remember up to a hundred other chickens, even after considerable time has passed.

And yes, unlike most birds, chickens like being cuddled by humans—certainly more than they like to be killed by them. In the United States alone, we slaughter nine *billion* chickens per year.

# EVERY TIME YOU
# BUY CHICKEN,
# YOU HURT A FARMER

Meet Jennifer Barrett of the Barrett Farm in Wickes, Arkansas. She and her husband, Rodney, are—were—third-generation chicken farmers. We thought you should hear directly from them because so many people we've talked to believe that farmers will suffer if consumers stop buying meat, dairy, and eggs. We won't mention who their suppliers were, because we don't want them to get sued. But you would readily recognize the brand because it's in almost every supermarket across the country.

*Here it is from Jennifer:*
Hard work is inherent in farming. I believe farmers are endowed with a gift to love it. We rise before dawn and fall into bed each night with a sense of accomplishment and fulfillment. We wouldn't want to live any other way.

My husband, Rodney, and I entered farming when we were young adults, taking over my parents' poultry business and dreaming of a quiet farm life where we could remain connected to nature and raise our children with a love of the earth and respect for life. We believed that farming animals was foundational work. It was a good old American job that would contribute to the well-being of everyone.

However, raising animals for food turns out to be quite different from most people's image of it. Because of our country's giant food industry, farming has become enormously competitive. To compete, you have to "go big or go home." This means a huge investment on the part of the farmer. For us, it meant signing a contract with a multinational food corporation and borrowing one million dollars to build four chicken houses. The bank thus owned the farm and the company dictated our farming practices, providing the chickens and the feed while we provided everything else. At first it looked like a great deal. The company did all the marketing and distribution, provided us with the "product" to grow and the feed to grow it. We did the work and the investment was ours. This would allow us to live out our quiet lives in the country and, in the end, leave us with our own profitable business.

In retrospect, however, what we did was sign ourselves up for indentured servitude. Half of every check went to the bank to cover the mortgage and the other half went back into the farm. The cost was exorbitant. We were raising a hundred thousand chickens every fifty-two days. It took massive amounts of electricity to run the fans used for cooling and ventilation. It took massive amounts of propane to heat the houses in the winter. The chickens drank enormous amounts of water. The mountains of poop they left behind had to be removed. Each working part in the whole operation had to be maintained and frequently needed repair. And, the whole lot of it was heavily taxed and insured. All told, in nearly nineteen years of raising chickens, we never once saw a profit.

The work itself was ceaseless. Every day we'd strap respirators to our faces and walk into a dimly lit sea of putrid stench to find and remove the dead. And, every day, they were there. These birds who would live fewer than eight weeks would succumb to disease or to the crushing weight of their disproportionate, genetically mutated bodies. Often they dropped dead from heart attacks due to their extreme rate of growth. Rodney culled the sick and injured chickens. He killed them by breaking their necks with a standard procedure prescribed by the company. It was imperative to the performance of the flock to keep the houses as "clean" as possible, which meant removing any inferior chickens.

> **"Half of every check went to the bank to cover the mortgage and the other half went back into the farm."**

The physical demands on our bodies and the constant financial stress took its toll. Our health began to decline because of our lifestyle and the endless financial worry. Our bright hopes of a quiet farm life became an inescapable nightmare.

In an effort to seek better health for ourselves, in 2016 we adopted a whole-food plant-based diet. We were astonished and somewhat perplexed to learn that we could thrive without any animal protein. This nugget of truth drove the severity of our situation to an even more desperate place. We had believed that all of our adversity was just the price a farmer paid to provide food. Learning that animal protein was optional nearly drove me mad. I couldn't understand why any of this hellish work or outrageous use of resources even existed.

It only exists because of market demand.

■ ■ ■

Jennifer and Rodney are not alone. Eating chicken doesn't just hurt chickens: It hurts the farmers who grow them. With the meteoric rise of fast-food chains like Chick-fil-A and Popeyes, small farms (which are overwhelmingly under corporate control) are struggling with America's insatiable appetite for chicken. Meanwhile, big-box retailers like Costco are in an arms race to sell the cheapest rotisserie chicken—now below $5 in many places. All of this means farmers are paid less and less to grow more and more chickens in horrendous conditions.

As NPR reported, "poultry growers often sign contracts for one flock at a time, with no guarantee that there will be another. They are also typically paid according to a tournament system: The best farmers are paid extra, with money taken away from farmers at the bottom."[75] Many farms take out multimillion-dollar loans to build the required infrastructure with no guarantee they will make their money back.

This kind of farming simply isn't sustainable—for the planet, for the farmers, and for the chickens themselves.

# COWS LOVE
# CLASSICAL MUSIC

Just like pigs and chickens, cows are much more intelligent than most people realize. They create complex social orders, they understand cause-and-effect relationships (a sign of advanced cognitive abilities), they keep friendships with their besties for life (when given the chance), and have unusually powerful mother–calf relationships. And, yes, like pigs, like humans, like individuals in any species, some may be a little dumber than others.

Most of this isn't surprising to those who have spent time with animals. What has surprised even bovinophiles is cows' elegant taste in music. In 2014, musicians from the Cleveland Orchestra visited Woodstock Farm Sanctuary in New York to see if rescued cows had any interest in classical music.[76] The moment the music started, a shy cow named Maybelle immediately shuffled toward the musicians and was soon joined by her friends, who were particularly fond of the oboe and violin. Want more? Search online for "cows love classical music" and watch the dozens of videos.

Scientists have studied the relationship between cows and music. For example, researchers at England's University of Leicester played various songs to herds of dairy cows to see if the music would improve their milk yield. The music alternated among silence, fast music, and slow music. The results? Cows wouldn't enjoy clubbing. They vastly preferred the slow music, from Simon & Garfunkel's "Bridge Over Troubled Water" to Beethoven's *Pastoral* Symphony—and, when that was played, they produced 3 percent more milk. Now, just think how much more they would enjoy the music if they weren't forced to be continuously pregnant and producing milk.

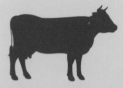

## BOVINE BESTIES:

**Cows create complex social orders, they understand cause-and-effect, and they maintain friendships for life.**

# YOU CAN HAVE
# YOUR BURGER
# AND EAT IT, TOO

Being vegan doesn't mean you have to live on salads and grain bowls (unless you're good with that). And it certainly doesn't mean you have to relinquish the decadent pleasure of wolfing down a burger with a side of fries. There are tons of great tasting, protein-rich vegan burgers. Like Beyond Meat says, its burger "looks, cooks, and satisfies like beef!"

So, go ahead: Forget for a night the responsible choices you should be making. Forget about eating purely unprocessed foods or getting the right nutrients. Sometimes you just need that deliciously wicked combo of fat, protein, and salt to make your dopamine receptors sing, and there are plenty of options for you.

So, indulge. If you want to make a burger at home, try:

- Beyond Meat
- Impossible Burger
- Hungry Planet
- Gardein
- Boca Burger
- Morningstar Farms
- Field Roast
- Amy's
- Dr. Praeger's (healthier)
- Sunshine Burgers (healthier)

Grab some vegan cheese (Daiya, Violife, and Follow Your Heart have excellent sliced cheese for sandwiches and burgers); add tomatoes and onions; slice up some avocado; dress it with ketchup, mustard, or relish; put all that goodness on a bun; and voila, it's like nothing ever changed.

And if you're out, there are many fast-food/fast-casual restaurants that have reliable vegan options, too. Every day there are more, so keep an eye out for your favorite places that may have recently added something to their menus. (We're not even listing foods like tacos and fried "chicken" because we're focusing on burgers, but there's an abundance of other meaty vegan offerings out there to satisfy every munchie whim.) If you want a fancier burger, ever more restaurants are featuring their own versions of a plant-based burger along with their animal-based fare; just call ahead to see what they have. If they don't have a vegan burger, ask to speak with the chef or manager so they can get with the program.

See? You don't have to miss out on anything, least of all the beloved burger.

# THERE'S NO NEED
# TO SPEND ON
# SUPPLEMENTS

Back in September 2019, news outlets breathlessly reported the story of an especially picky eater who subsisted on a robust diet of French fries, Pringles potato chips, white bread, and processed pork. By the age of seventeen, thanks to a complete lack of essential vitamins, he had suffered severe damage to his optic nerve and was declared legally blind, despite being prescribed a heavy battery of nutritional supplements. The boy was even the subject of a case study in the *Annals of Internal Medicine*: "Blindness Caused by a Junk Food Diet."[77]

As this unfortunate case proved, no amount of supplements can make up for a poor diet. In fact, "Not only are vitamin and mineral supplements a waste of money, they can in some instances actually harm the body," reported *The Guardian* in 2018, after researchers from the University of Toronto published a meta-analysis of all randomized controlled trials that examined the effects of supplements on heart disease and stroke risk. It turns out that the most commonly popped supplements—multivitamins, calcium, and vitamin C—seem to provide no health benefits. And taking some vitamins, such as $B_3$, A, C, and E, was even associated with increased mortality rates. How about calcium?

A 2011 study in *The BMJ* found that calcium supplements "modestly increase the risk of cardio-vascular events," including heart attack and stroke.[78] Moreover, a study published in *The American Journal of Clinical Nutrition* reported "no reduction in hip fracture risk with calcium supplementation, and an increased risk is possible."[79]

Fish oil supplements, meanwhile, are one of the most commonly taken supplements, with nearly 19 million US adults and children throwing them back regularly.[80] The idea goes that fish such as anchovies, bluefish, herring, and mackerel are naturally high in omega-3 fatty acids, which have been shown to decrease your risk of heart disease by lowering triglyceride levels. So by killing a lot of fish and compressing their oil into pills, can you truly ward off disease? Three massive studies from 2019 certainly aren't on board. The first, published in *The BMJ*, found that fish supplements had little to no benefit for diabetes patients trying to lower blood-glucose levels. The next study, published in the *Annals of Internal Medicine*, had a "low level of certainty" that omega-3 supplements did anything to ward off coronary heart disease after sifting through data from nearly a million patients. Finally, an analysis published in the *New England Journal of Medicine* tracking twenty-six thousand people concluded that fish oil was completely useless when it came to preventing invasive breast, prostate, or colorectal cancer.[81]

The best way to take in your essential vitamins and minerals? According to the same researchers quoted above, it's "by getting vitamins and minerals from a healthy diet, which includes lots of fruit and vegetables." Plants contain all seventeen of the major and minor essential minerals, which come from the soil, are incorporated into the plant tissue, and cling to roots, stems, and leaves. Whether you're eating spinach, broccoli, beans, or just about any other plant, you're getting a healthy dose of essential minerals straight from the source. As for vitamins, eleven out of thirteen are readily available in plant foods. The exceptions are vitamin D, which comes from the sun, and vitamin $B_{12}$, which comes from microorganisms in the soil. If you don't spend a lot of time in the sun, your doctor may suggest a vitamin D supplement—or you could simply help yourself to the wide assortment of vitamin D–fortified plant foods such as nut milks and whole-grain cereals.

There is a lot of misinformation about $B_{12}$, a crucial vitamin that helps build red blood cells and DNA. Your body does not synthesize it on its own, so you have to ingest it through diet. Contrary to what your paleo friends might tell you, animal products are not the only source of vitamin $B_{12}$; rather, it's produced by bacteria in the earth.[82] Early humans had no problem getting enough $B_{12}$ because they ate berries, roots, and other tough vegetables caked in soil. Cows typically get $B_{12}$ from the dirt-covered grass, chickens ingest it while pecking for worms and other insects, and a small amount is passed to humans who eat their flesh. The present-day water we drink is purified and our produce is heavily washed, so we need more help getting enough $B_{12}$, typically through a supplement or fortified foods.

For most people, two 1,000 mcg $B_{12}$ supplements twice per week is sufficient, but be sure to check with your doctor first.

# BEANS HELP YOU LIVE LONGER

Humans are obsessed with extending their life span—understandable, since death is, well, kind of scary.

In Christian teachings, the cup Jesus drank from during the Last Supper was later used by Joseph of Arimathea to catch his blood on the cross. Since then, everyone from crusading knights to Indiana Jones has looked for this Holy Grail because of its purported ability to heal wounds and grant eternal life. Two thousand years after Jesus, the heirs of baseball great Ted Williams cryogenically froze the left fielder's remains shortly after his death, hoping that resurrection technology may one day be available. In recent years, the ultra-wealthy have reportedly pioneered the practice of "young blood transfusions," in which older people inject themselves with the blood of younger, healthier people in hopes of slowing the aging process.

For the rest of us, who don't have millions of dollars lying around to freeze our bodies or harvest blood from teenagers, there's a cheaper, safer, and monumentally less creepy way to live longer: Eat beans.

The lowly bean doesn't get much respect. Many people avoid them because they're afraid of increased flatulence (more on that on page 125). And, admittedly, their presentation isn't all that great: They come in cans (unless you're a culinary badass and buy them uncooked, which you definitely should try doing because they are so hearty and delish), they look kind of earth-toned, and they're just, well . . . beans. Lots of superfoods have exotic names like acai berries, spirulina, mangosteen, and cacao. Kidney beans, on the other hands, sound a lot less sexy. We get it—beans are boring. But their health effects are anything but.

First things first: What exactly are beans? Technically speaking, beans are classified into a broader category of plant foods called *legumes*. Most of the legumes you're familiar with can be further classified as *pulses*. Here are some of the most common forms of pulses at the grocery store:

- Beans: black, pinto, kidney, black-eyed peas, fava

- Chickpeas (garbanzo beans)

- Dry peas: whole green, split green, whole yellow, split yellow

- Lentils: green, black, brown, red

For the purposes of this book, let's keep things simple and call all of the above *beans*. Just like vegetables, beans are full of healthy vitamins, minerals, fiber, and phytonutrients. But they also pack in large amounts of clean protein, which makes them uniquely situated in the Plant Food Hall of Fame. And it just so happens that these unassuming little guys can add years to your life span.

If you won't take it from us, take it from the American Institute for Cancer Research, which published the most comprehensive study of diet and cancer ever in 2007. After analyzing some five hundred thousand studies, nine research teams reached a conclusion about which foods could most effectively prevent cancer. Drumroll . . . it's beans![83] And not just every week or day, but every meal! It turns out the English were right: You *should* have beans for breakfast (though maybe lay off the bacon, fried bread, and sausages).

> **The single best supplement you can take every day to live longer is a cup of beans.**

Beans are jam-packed with nutrition. For instance, a mere 3.5-ounce serving of chickpeas delivers 18 percent of your daily protein, 30 percent of your daily fiber, and 43 percent of your daily folate. That goes along with no cholesterol, and only trace amounts of fat and sodium.

There's perhaps no one better to consult about longevity than National Geographic fellow and author of *The Blue Zones*, Dan Buettner. Put simply, Blue Zones are the five places in the world where people live the longest: Okinawa, Japan; the Nicoya Peninsula of Costa Rica; the highlands of Sardinia; Loma Linda, California; and Ikaria, Greece. After studying these populations for years, Dan says the single best supplement you can take every day to live longer is a cup of beans: cheap, humble beans. He calculates that if eaten regularly, these nuggets of nutrition can add about four years to your life. This supremely simple food is a daily dish throughout all the Blue Zones, whether it's

## FART FACT: YOUR FARTS WILL SMELL LIKE PERFUME

Okay, fine, maybe your farts won't smell like Chanel No. 5. But they'll certainly smell a lot better on a vegan diet.

Let's clear the air about the old myth that eating lots of beans will cause you to clear a room with noxious bodily fumes. While everyone should be eating as many lentils, black beans, kidney beans, pinto beans, and chickpeas as possible, many don't because they are afraid about increased gas.

Well, here's some good news: Fear of farts is just a load of hot air.

Believe it or not, there have been quite a few scientific analyses of beans and farting. For instance, in a study helpfully titled "Perceptions of Flatulence from Bean Consumption Among Adults in 3 Feeding Studies" and published in the *Nutrition Journal*, researchers asked a group of brave participants to eat a half cup of beans daily and respond to a questionnaire. Did these bean-eaters clear out subway cars with their atomic flatulence? Nope. It turns out that, "in the first week, fewer than half of the bean eaters reported increases in gas production." In fact, "seventy percent or more of the participants who experienced flatulence felt that it dissipated by the second or third week of bean consumption."[84] So, once your body adjusts to a high-fiber diet, your flatulence fears will dissipate like a you-know-what in the wind.

Concerned more about the quality of your farts than the quantity? Good news: That fart odor mainly comes from foods high in sulfur, namely seafood, eggs, and meat.

in the minestrone of Sardinia or the hummus in Loma Linda or the tofu in Okinawa. Dan says the secret to making them a part of your daily diet is to learn how to make them delicious, and we highly recommend his cookbook, *The Blue Zones Kitchen*, to help you do just that.

Some of you Iron Chefs out there might prefer to cook raw beans, and we don't blame you. Aside from the familiars, there are so many heirloom varieties to try, such as Christmas, Cranberry, and Eye of the Goat beans. They may take hours to cook depending on what method you use, but you might try a pressure cooker if you're not cool with minding the stove. Home-cooked beans are generally tastier than canned beans, and they're also cheaper because you can buy in bulk. But for some of us, precooked canned beans are perfectly fine. If possible, opt for low-sodium products, and be sure to wash canned beans thoroughly; if you don't, the added sodium might cancel out the beans' heart-healthy effects.

# YOU CAN
# SAVE MONEY

The notion that eating vegan is expensive is absurd. The populations who eat a mostly plant-based diet—remember the Blue Zones (see page 124)—are hardly wealthy by any standards. Think of the shepherds living in the highlands of Sardinia, Italy; the farmers on the faraway island of Ikaria, Greece; or the people tending their land in Costa Rica's Nicoya Peninsula—all these groups tend to be simple people living within very modest means. Their diet consists mostly of beans, grains, and seasonal vegetables and fruits, along with some nuts and seeds. They enjoy thick soups with homemade sourdough bread, hearty pastas, a bounty of vegetable dishes, sweet potatoes and tofu, beans in everything, and maybe a little vino or sake at the end of the day. That stuff is simple and cheap, it fills you up while keeping you energized, and it keeps you healthy.

The staples of a vegan diet are cheap. Oatmeal is cheap. Peanut butter is cheap. Chickpeas and black beans are cheap. Tortillas and sweet potatoes are cheap. Hazelnuts and pumpkin seeds are cheap. Apples and bananas are affordable in season, while other fancier fruits can be purchased frozen (which is just as nutritious) at a really good price. We both buy our kale, broccoli, spinach, mangoes,

## VEGAN DIET STAPLES ARE CHEAP:

Oatmeal. Peanut butter.
Chickpeas and black
beans. Tortillas
and sweet potatoes.
Hazelnuts and
pumpkin seeds.

blueberries, strawberries, and peaches frozen, and throw huge handfuls into a daily smoothie for a regular hit of phytonutrients. And when it comes to more expensive items—say, plant-based yogurt, burgers, and cheeses—think of them as a luxury, not a necessity.

There's more. You will save more money in the long term, because you will be healthier. You'll have more energy to be creative and productive; you'll miss less work. You'll have fewer doctor bills.

And think what you'll do for society as a whole! You'll reduce the chances that you'll get heart disease, diabetes, cancer, and other costly chronic diseases—those expensive chronic diseases paid for by . . . us.

According to a report by the Alzheimer's Association, "From 2010 to 2050, the cost of caring for Americans 65 and older with Alzheimer's disease will increase more than six times to $1.08 trillion. Currently, $172 billion a year is spent by the government, private insurance and individuals to care for people with the disease, the most common cause of dementia."[85] (For more about the link between diet and dementia, see page 172.)

Heart disease costs more than $500 billion annually, yet it's almost entirely preventable with a plant-based diet. And cancer? More than $225 billion. Type 2 diabetes? About $175 billion, and it's also almost completely preventable. Think about all the wonderful things the country could afford by thwarting these debilitating conditions in the first place through healthier plant-based food choices.

# PLANT FOODS =
## ZERO CHOLESTEROL

Here's another fun fact: Dietary cholesterol is found *only* in animal foods.

Before we dive deeper into that, let's briefly recap: Cholesterol is a waxy substance that your body uses to build new cells. Your body can't live without it, which is why your handy-dandy liver pumps out all the cholesterol you need. The problems arise when there is too much cholesterol—specifically LDL, the "bad" cholesterol—in your blood, which joins with other substances to create hard deposits along your artery walls, called plaque. The long-term narrowing of your arteries reduces blood flow and damages the heart; if a chunk of plaque breaks off and a blood clot forms, you may have a heart attack, perhaps a fatal one.

As we saw earlier, eating foods containing lots of saturated and trans fats (primarily from animal foods) causes your liver to pump out more LDL cholesterol. But here's the double whammy: The same animal products also contain ready-made cholesterol, known as dietary cholesterol. In other words, not only are animal products chock-full of the building blocks—saturated and trans fats—that work together to raise your cholesterol level, they contain premade, fully armed and operational cholesterol ready to wreak havoc on your body. Take eggs, for example. If you look at the nutrition label, you'll see a mere 1.6 grams of saturated fat. That may not seem so bad . . . until you see that it also has 187 mg of dietary cholesterol. (For more about eggs, see page 46.)

Need proof? In 2019, researchers from Northwestern Medicine in Chicago reported that adults who consumed the most dietary cholesterol had a significantly higher risk of death, especially from cardiovascular disease. "The take-home message is really about cholesterol, which happens to be high in eggs and specifically yolks," explained a lead researcher. "As part of a healthy diet, people need to consume lower amounts of cholesterol. People who consume less cholesterol have a lower risk of heart disease."[86]

**"Plants are . . . rich in soluble fiber, which helps lower cholesterol."**

Plant foods are exactly the opposite: They contain zero dietary cholesterol. As the Physicians Committee for Responsible Medicine explains, "They are very low in saturated fat and free of cholesterol. Plants are also rich in soluble fiber, which helps lower cholesterol. Soluble fiber slows the absorption of cholesterol and reduces the amount of cholesterol the liver produces."[87]

# 5 0

# THOSE TERRIBLE TRANS FATS ARE STILL AROUND

Remember trans fats? Those nutritional bad boys that have been linked to higher LDL cholesterol levels and heart disease? They're those freaky fat molecules created when food manufacturers make liquid oils creamy. By the early 2000s, basically everyone agreed that trans fats are absolutely horrible for our health and should be banned. California and New York City were among the first to banish hydrogenated oils from restaurants in the mid-2000s. At long last, in 2013, the Food and Drug Administration determined that trans fats are not "generally recognized as safe"—government mumbo jumbo for "they must be removed from the food supply."

And while it's true that there are, generally speaking, no more foods prepared with trans fats (even the few stragglers—some frozen pizzas, sweet pies, and chips—that were given permission to use trans fats until they figured out a healthier replacement ingredient have almost entirely been phased out), it's still worth checking the ingredients labels for "partially hydrogenated" oils.

Sounds like everything is moving in the right direction. But for this: The FDA has banned only *artificial* trans fats. That's because in their natural form, these ne'er-do-wells come straight from Mother Nature. Trans fat is found in the meat and dairy from ruminant animals, that is, cows, sheep, and goats. So, if you eat meat, you are eating trans fat. There's no avoiding it. And if you think that these trace amounts of trans fat aren't a big deal, take it from the Harvard Medical School: "Even small amounts of trans fats can harm health: For every 2 percent of calories from trans fat consumed daily, the risk of heart disease rises by 23 percent."[88]

Some of your meat-eating friends will still argue that natural trans fat is different from artificial trans fat. If that was the case, why did the National Academy of Sciences (NAS), perhaps the most prestigious scientific organization in the country, conclude that there is no safe level of *any* form of trans fat? "Any incremental increase in trans fatty acid intake increases coronary heart disease risk," a NAS report explained.[89] A 2012 study published in the *British Nutrition Journal* confirmed that trans fat from animals is still very bad for human health, especially among women.[90]

The NAS concluded in its report that "because trans fats are unavoidable on ordinary, nonvegan diets, getting down to 0 percent trans fats would require significant changes in patterns of dietary intake." That's government speak for: "Stop eating meat and dairy!"

# TYPE 2 DIABETES IS NOT ABOUT CARBS. IT'S ABOUT FAT.

Type 2 diabetes is an epidemic. More than one-third of the US population either suffers from it or its precursor, prediabetes, and about 463 million adults are living with it worldwide, according to the International Diabetes Federation.[91] That number is predicted to rise to 700 million by 2045.

Not only does diabetes lead to some four million deaths each year, it's also extremely expensive to treat. According to the American Diabetes Association, the estimated total direct and indirect costs of diabetes in the United States in 2017 was $327 billion.[92] And globally, the bill comes close to $760 billion USD.

**When you eat fat it builds up in the cells of your muscles and liver.**

You may have heard that the cause of this epidemic is carbs, but that's not true. Yes, cookies and cake will make things worse, but the real culprit is fat. When you eat fat—especially the saturated fat from animal foods—it builds up in the cells of your muscles and liver. The job of insulin is to shuttle glucose (made from carbohydrates) into the cells where it can be turned into fuel for your body. But if there is a buildup of fat inside your cells, insulin can't access your cells, meaning all that extra glucose lingers in your blood, causing your blood sugar to skyrocket to dangerous levels. The buildup of glucose in your blood is known officially as insulin resistance, and it's the cause of type 2 diabetes. To avoid it (and thus diabetes), steer clear of fatty animal foods. It's that easy.

And yet, many doctors tell their diabetic and prediabetic patients to avoid carbs and starchy vegetables—a terrible mistake since whole grains, potatoes, fruits, and vegetables are packed with fiber, which slows down the release of glucose so that it doesn't overwhelm your cells' ability to absorb it. So there's no need to demonize starchy foods! If you are diabetic or prediabetic, talk to your doctor first, of course, but avoid processed carbs like white rice, pasta, and snack foods, while incorporating delicious brown rice, quinoa, and other whole grains. And keep that gummy fat out of your cells by opting for naturally low-fat, plant-based foods.

# YOU CAN BE
# VEGANISH

T ake. Your. Time. You can just transition to a vegan diet at a pace that's comfortable. Explore new foods, different restaurants, and fresh recipes. There are lots of ways to do this. Follow Instagrammers who inspire your journey. Meet up with people who share your curiosity or are further along in their plant-based progression. If you feel socially awkward at a party or holiday dinner because you're the only one not dipping into the meaty stuff, just remember that you're not bonkers for wanting to eat healthier or for caring about the planet and/or animals. (And, seriously, who cares if someone ribs you for avoiding the ribs?)

Be proud to be out front. What may be strange or different now will most certainly be common in another decade, so embrace your status as an early adopter. Don't be a twit and lecture your friends, but take a minute to appreciate the fact that you are doing right by your body and helping to make the world a better place. If people don't like it, that's cool; that's their right, just like it's your right to keep growing and changing. Smile and be kind, especially to yourself. This is a process. You and your family and friends have probably been eating animals for generations, so you're not going to shift overnight without the occasional hiccup.

That's why starting slowly makes this way of eating stick; you find your footing, get your game on, and then you're off and running.

Oh, and perfectionism—we're not into that. There's no contest for who can be the most or best vegan. Vegan*ish* is just fine. You don't have to drive the waiter crazy with questions about whether there's egg in the bread. If he says it's egg-free, believe him and move on. If you're at a party and you're starving and you're eyeballing cheese and crackers because there's absolutely nothing non-animal to eat, have it. The vegan mafia won't come for you. Over the next week, put some energy into finding a great vegan cheese that you like, and bring it to the party next time. Share your goodies; people love a good food find!

Life is meant to be enjoyed, and food is a big part of that. So much of our comfort and pleasure is connected to enjoying traditional favorites with our peeps. Advice: Continue to enjoy what you grew up loving; just upgrade it a little so it's better for your body and soul. Do you love sausage in your pasta? Great, try your favorite recipe with one of the new brands of

> **The vegan mafia won't come for you.**

animal-free meat. Like tostadas and burritos? No problem. Use beans instead of beef or chicken, and pile on the guac and salsa. Wine and cheese for happy hour is your favorite thing in life? Make a spread with vegan cheese or hummus and toast your progress. A latte on your way to work? Oat milk is the greatest thing since oatmeal. Turkey or lamb on holidays? Keep it healthy with a lentil loaf or, better yet, indulge with a plant-based alternative to whatever meat you've been accustomed to. This is not about white-knuckle, hard-core discipline; it's about finding the foods that work for your life and keep you happy.

We hope you feel so good that you want to go all the way eventually. Maybe you'll get there—or maybe you'll get close enough. Once the door is open, you'll likely just keep leaning forward and exploring. Trust yourself to take the next right step.

You already have.

**ADVICE:**

**Continue to enjoy what you grew up loving; just upgrade it a little so it's better for your body and soul.**

# BECAUSE BABIES!

Thinking about having a baby? Not surprisingly, diet plays a major role in a woman's ability to get and stay pregnant. Certain key vitamins and minerals support healthy functioning of the reproductive system, particularly folic acid, iron, omega-3 fatty acids, and zinc. Low amounts of these nutrients can decrease fertility. What is the best source of these Vs&Ms?

An eight-year study that examined the eating patterns of tens of thousands of women who were trying to conceive revealed that women who ate predominantly plant-based foods were found to lower their risk of problems during ovulation by two-thirds and other infertility risks by more than a quarter.[93]

Here are some Dietary Dos and Don'ts if you're planning to get pregnant:

- Load up on vegetables and other produce. Besides providing antioxidants and other compounds that fight inflammation and free radical damage, these fibrous, healthy carbs also keep blood sugar in check. Lower levels of all three are linked to better fertility.

- For the same reasons, get protein from lentils, chickpeas, nuts, and other plant sources.

- Ditto iron: Eat leafy greens, not steak.

- Add more healthy fats like olive oil and avocados while avoiding inflammatory animal-based saturated and especially trans fats.

Other research backs up vegan-friendly diets. A recent Australian study found that the more fruit women ate, and the less junk food they scarfed down, the more easily they became pregnant. And additives like artificial hormones fed to farm animals, along with contaminants like mercury, dioxins, and other pollutants stored in fish and mammal fat, have been found to wreak havoc on human hormones necessary for fertility.

**FERTILE FACT:** While most of the evidence favoring a plant-based diet applies to mothers-to-be, a growing body of research shows that a healthy vegan lifestyle also supports the production and quality of a man's sperm.

# BEING VEGAN CAN
# MAKE YOU HAPPIER

Feeling dark? Before you go all in on Prozac, try going plant.

Recent research indicates that plants can lift your spirits—in part because of their ample antioxidants, which help protect the body and brain from inflammation, which can negatively influence mood and energy levels and interfere with the brain's self-repair process. Skipping the steak also helps you skirt the damaging effects of a compound called arachidonic acid, which is found in animal foods and is linked to brain inflammation.

Additionally, a growing body of research finds a strong link between gut health (see page 73) and emotional stability. The nutrients in plants support a happy microbiome filled with friendly bacteria, whereas meat introduces harmful microbes. Recent studies show participants who cut meat from their diets saw not just a rapid change in their gut bacteria, but also a corresponding improvement in their mood and outlook.

Certain spices and seeds also seem to have mood-elevating qualities, notably saffron, which has been shown to work as well as the antidepressant drug Prozac in the treatment of clinical depression—without the side effects.[94] Likewise, scientists have tested sesame, sunflower, and pumpkin seeds for their efficacy in treating social anxiety disorder, all of which have been shown, in research doctor language, to bring "significant improvement in an objective measurement in anxiety within an hour of consumption."

Dr. Drew Ramsey, a Columbia University psychiatrist who studies the link between diet patterns and mental health conditions, found that low levels of twelve nutrients—including omega-3 fatty acids, B vitamins, vitamin D, iron, magnesium, and zinc—can be linked to depressive symptoms, and that replenishing them helps prevent or relieve these symptoms. In his study ranking foods by "antidepressant nutrient score," expressed as a percentage, the top scorers were plants, especially leafy greens, pumpkin, and peppers. With the exception of oysters, no animal foods scored nearly as high as plants. And while key vitamins $B_{12}$ and $D_3$ aren't found in plants, vegans consume the former in fortified foods or a supplement and get the latter by spending time in the sun.

**Plants, with their ample antioxidants, help protect the body and brain from inflammation.**

And, of course there's this: Unlike meat-eaters, vegans don't suffer from the stress and guilt that comes from thinking about the cruel factory farming of the animals who became their pork chops and chicken wings. Sorry. Had to throw that in.

# CROWDING OUT
# FOOD IS EASIER THAN
# CUTTING OUT FOOD

Most diets have you cutting out foods; they are about denial and discipline. (Translation: Diets are boring, annoying, and impossible to maintain for most people.) But eating vegan is not a fad diet; it's a shift toward conscious eating that should bring you happiness and joy, not gloom and boredom.

This is why we recommend "crowding out, not cutting out," meaning that you *add* enough nutrient-rich, fiber-filled plant foods to your diet that, before you know it, you don't have the belly space to squeeze in the old earth-damaging, health-threatening foods. When you've eaten a handful of pistachios here and a couple of peaches there, when you've allowed fiber-rich food to fill you up (while bringing your blood sugar under control), you're not at the mercy of wild cravings to eat something, anything, for a temporary boost of energy. And you're going to start feeling so freaking good you'll want to keep that vibe going.

Try thinking about it this way: As soon as someone says you shouldn't have a steak, all you're going to think about is that steak you shouldn't have. You'll be drawn to it because it's brought you satisfaction before (along with a possible coronary incident). Instead of trying to resist your craving, tell yourself that you can have whatever you want, but first you're going to have some hummus or fruit. (And water, because sometimes we think we're hungry when we're actually thirsty.)

We also are big believers in switching up your favorite dishes to plant-based versions so that you don't slip into thoughts like "Poor me, I can never have pizza again" or "Pancakes are the light of my life and I simply can't live without them." The answer is to just veganize what you already love. If pizza owns your heart, pick up a pizza crust at the grocery store or order some online, spread out the tomato sauce, sprinkle on some vegan cheese, add a few dollops of whatever other plant-based toppings you want (vegan sausage is crazy good, by the way), and pop your creation into the oven. Of course, you can also google "vegan pizza near me" if you want to go out.

If your weakness is pancakes, crowd out the ones your mom made with eggs and butter and make them with oatmeal, flax, and banana to create some of the best flapjacks you've ever had. (There are tons of recipes online, just look for "vegan oatmeal pancakes.") The point is that anything you're used to enjoying, you can still enjoy . . . just crowd out the animal-based ingredients with cleaner, animal-free ones. Boom, everyone's happy.

This kind of tweaking will nudge you away from what may have seemed like the unshakable habits of eating animal stuff. Other shifts will follow, but you can implement them when you're good and ready. Eating vegan should never be a chore, but rather a cool adventure.

Use these plant-based ingredients to crowd out animal-based ones:

- Flaxseed meal, chia, agar (seaweed), applesauce, or egg replacer instead of eggs in baked goods

- Oat, soy, almond, hemp, or rice milk instead of cow's milk

- Olive or coconut oil or vegan butter instead of butter

- Hummus, avocado, or vegan mayo instead of mayo made with eggs

- Lentils/beans, jackfruit, or plant-based meat instead of ground beef or chicken

- Thinly sliced tempeh instead of bacon

- Chickpea spread instead of tuna

- Wild mushrooms, tofu, or seitan instead of meat

- Plant-based yogurt instead of goat or cow's milk yogurt

- Nutritional yeast instead of parmesan

- Scrambled tofu with turmeric instead of scrambled eggs

- Aquafaba (chickpea brine) instead of eggs for meringue

- Cashew cream instead of dairy cream

- Agave or maple syrup instead of honey

# Vegan Pancakes

*Enjoy these amazing, fluffy pancakes with vegan butter and warm maple syrup, or change things up and serve with sliced fresh fruit. You can also stir into the batter your choice of fruit (blueberries or sliced bananas are great), chopped nuts, or dark chocolate chips. This recipe is courtesy of our friend Robin Robertson, one of the best vegan cookbook authors around.*

1½ cups unbleached all-purpose flour

3 tablespoons natural sugar

1 tablespoon baking powder

¼ teaspoon sea salt

2 tablespoons ground golden flaxseeds

¼ cup warm water

1¼ cups almond milk or other plant milk

2 teaspoons apple cider vinegar

1 teaspoon pure vanilla extract

Cooking spray for griddle

Warm maple syrup and vegan butter, to serve

**1** In a large bowl, combine the flour, sugar, baking powder, and salt. Mix well and set aside.

**2** In a medium bowl, combine the flaxseeds and warm water, stirring to blend well. Add the almond milk, vinegar, and vanilla and blend until smooth.

**3** Pour the wet ingredients into the dry ingredients, mixing until just combined. Do not overmix. The batter should be thick. A few small lumps are okay.

**4** Heat a griddle or large nonstick skillet over medium heat and coat it lightly with cooking spray. For each pancake, ladle about ¼ cup of batter onto the hot griddle. Make as many pancakes at once that will fit on the griddle or skillet without touching.

**5** Cook the pancakes on one side until small bubbles appear on top, about 3 minutes. Flip the pancakes with a metal spatula and cook until the other side is lightly browned, about 2 minutes longer. Repeat until all the batter has been used. Serve hot with warm maple syrup and vegan butter.

**MAKES 4 SERVINGS**

# YOU CAN LOWER
# YOUR BODY FAT

I f you are overweight, your doctor might have told you to lower your BMI (Body Mass Index), which is a ratio of your height to your weight (technically, for the math geeks out there, it's your weight in kilograms divided by your height in meters squared). Very generally speaking, you want your BMI to fall between 18.5 and 24.9, although this calculation does not account for conditioned athletes, bone density, fat distribution, and other variables. No matter what your BMI is, if you are attempting to cut some excess body fat, you don't have to begin a restrictive diet. Quite the contrary: You can eat nearly all the food you want as long as that food is whole and plant-based.

According to a report published in *PLOS ONE* (a journal of the Public Library of Science) in 2018 that examined the results of 40 different studies, a plant-based diet reduces BMI. Another research effort, published in 2013 in the *Journal of the Academy of Nutrition and Dietetics*, found that, among study participants, BMI was lowest among vegans, while the average BMI was highest among meat-eaters. And, in a study longwindedly referred to as the Oxford cohort of the European Prospective Investigation into Cancer and Nutrition (EPIC-Oxford), the conclusion was the following: "Fish-eaters, vegetarians and especially vegans had lower

BMI than meat-eaters. . . . High protein and low fibre intakes were the factors most strongly associated with increasing BMI."[95]

So, why count calories to reduce your weight when all you have to do is eat a healthy, whole-food, vegan diet?

## NO NEED FOR A RESTRICTIVE DIET:

You can eat nearly all the food you want as long as that food is whole and plant-based.

# GOOD GENES
# NEED PLANTS

Anyone who tells you that your health is simply a matter of good genes versus bad genes hasn't read the work done by Dr. Dean Ornish and Nobel Prize–winner Elizabeth Blackburn, PhD. These two scientists, both highly respected in their fields, found that a vegan diet caused more than 500 genes to change their expression in only three months.[96] In other words, your body can potentially activate dormant genes that help prevent disease, while turning off genes that cause breast cancer, heart disease, prostate cancer, and other chronic illnesses.

Translation: Just because your daddy and his daddy before him got diabetes does not mean you will too. You have the power, through better diet, to stave off what's been lurking in your family line.

Dean Ornish first showed back in the mid-1990s that heart disease is reversible by making comprehensive lifestyle changes, which include shifting to a plant-based diet, managing stress, and getting regular (but modest) exercise. Even severe coronary heart disease can be reversed when you make these healthy upgrades to your daily routine.

Elizabeth Blackburn is a molecular biologist and biochemist who discovered that telomeres, the caps at the end of your DNA strands, protect our chromosomes from damage. Unfortunately, they tend to get shorter as we age, accelerating the aging (aka dying) process. The question was: Do our telomeres automatically shorten with age, or do we get some say in the process?

Dr. Blackburn, working with Dr. Ornish, studied men with low-grade prostate cancer, watching what happened to patients who made Dr. Ornish's lifestyle changes compared with the ones who simply kept eating and doing what they always had. The researchers reported that the men who shifted to a predominantly plant-based diet actually *lengthened* their telomeres by 10 percent. The men who kept on keeping on with the Standard American Diet? Their poor telomeres were 3 percent shorter on average.[97]

**You have the power, through better diet, to stave off what's been lurking in your family line.**

Drs. Blackburn and Ornish determined that the foods that shorten telomeres are red meat, white bread, sweetened drinks, saturated fat, soda, and excessive alcohol. The foods associated with longer telomeres? Whole grains, vegetables, nuts, beans, seaweed, fruits, and coffee.

So no, it's not all in your genes. A lot of it is on your plate.

# SPENT DAIRY
# COWS BECOME
# HAMBURGERS
# AND DOG FOOD

f there's anyone in the world you don't want to be, it's a dairy cow. As we know, mothers produce milk when they have babies, and shortly after a baby calf is born, it is snatched away from the mother, because the milk is designated for people, not the calf nature intended it for. The mother cow naturally goes bananas, because there's nothing more painful—in any species—than for a mother to lose her offspring. The baby can barely walk, so she's carted away. The mom bellows in anguish for days, calling for her calf, bucking if she has the space, and sometimes knocking her head against anything she can find.

Right after giving birth, the mother is hooked up to a milking machine several times a day every day, with hard metal that clamps on to her teats, and it pulls and sucks at her until she's dry. She stands on hard metal slats, which eventually causes her to go lame. As we saw in reason 5 (see page 17), because she's usually dosed with a bovine growth hormone, she may develop a painful infection in her udder called mastitis.

A cow should live up to 25 years, but a typical dairy cow will only live until the age of four or five because her body gets worn out after multiple births and constant milking. Once she is considered useless, she is loaded onto a truck (occasionally, as undercover footage has shown, via forklift, since she can no longer walk), and sent to the slaughterhouse to be turned into hamburgers or dog food.

**FRIGHTFUL FACT:** One beef patty can have the meat of up to 100 cows in it.

# MEAT IS THE
# NEW TOBACCO

If you watched the TV show *Mad Men*, or any movie set before the 1970s, chances are that your favorite stars were smoking like chimneys in just about every scene—before breakfast, at the office, before sex, after sex, in bed while reading, and so on. Few understood that they were effectively mainlining carcinogens into their bodies and, with every inhalation, damaging their lungs. This was all because the tobacco industry was hiding the truth from the world.

Today, we have a similar situation with meat.

Tobacco companies created a safe, pro-smoking image in ads depicting ruggedly handsome cowboys smoking while perched on their horses and glamorous, responsible-looking mothers sharing cigarettes with their gossip. But smoking wasn't just made to look cool, it was made to look healthy, too. (One of the most infamous phrases in advertising history has to be that cigarettes are "doctor recommended.") There were ads that touted smoking's weight-reducing effects, not to mention one that the cigarette giant Philip Morris ran featuring a physician who said, after prescribing cigarettes to patients with irritated throats (yes, *prescribing* cigarettes), "Every case of irritation cleared completely or definitely improved."[98]

The tobacco industry spent big money to create this facade of wholesomeness, and for decades the public bought in. Even after science had documented the deadly effects of tobacco, cigarette companies flooded the airwaves with pseudoscience claiming otherwise. They obfuscated ad nauseam. And people continued to smoke. Thanks to the addictive nature of tobacco products, nearly a billion people worldwide still do.[99] Yes, a billion.

Now think about how we've done an about-face on smoking, and how it all seems so obvious now. We may just be in that same beginning stage of a reversal on meat consumption: Today, doctors (most of whom receive very little nutrition training during medical school) tend to recommend you get ample protein through animal sources. Blogs and podcasts everywhere are touting the ways of the trendy (and deadly) keto diet (see page 38).

**The science has long since been in on how detrimental meat and dairy is.**

The science has long since been in on how detrimental meat and dairy is for us, and it's likely that animal food probably kills a lot more people than tobacco does. The biggest killers of our time—heart disease, stroke, diabetes, and certain cancers—are all linked to animal consumption, and people who eat a plant-based diet have much lower risks of all four.

Why aren't we hearing strong warnings to steer clear of animal food? Because just as with the

## THERE'S BIG MONEY IN MEAT:

If you're wondering about the validity of any study, look to see who funded it.

tobacco industry, there's big money in meat. And those special interests invest in "scientific" papers that twist the results to make it sound like meat, eggs, and dairy aren't so bad for you. If you're wondering about the validity of any study, look to see who funded it. If it's something supported by the National Egg Association or the Cattlemen's Beef Association, take a wild guess what the results of the study will show: Their product is healthy. How convenient!

Governmental institutions that directly influence policy, such as dietary guidelines that schools and medical institutions are supposed to follow, are presided over by lobbyists of major food producers. It's hard to find the real truth in all the pseudoscience that's out in the public domain, but fruits and vegetables do not have the same well-funded lobbyists twisting the dietary science, and they sure aren't causing obesity and heart disease. Big Broccoli and Big Kale are not out to swindle you into shopping in the produce aisle.

We're not yet at the point where bacon and eggs are seen as the health equivalent of smoking a pack of cigarettes, but we're getting there. Future generations will look back on how we ate animal foods and wonder, "What were they thinking?" just like we look at our grandparents and wonder how in the world they thought it was okay to smoke three packs per day.

# THE MEAT BUSINESS
# COSTS YOU MONEY

66 I 'd love to go vegan . . . but it's just too expensive!" We've heard this old chestnut more times than we can count. Somehow, over the years, we've been indoctrinated with the fallacy that plant-based food is prohibitively expensive. As we saw on page 127, eating plant-based is very budget-friendly as long as you know how to shop. But it is also true that, at least at the cash register, meat is cheap, too. You can get chunks of beef or a chicken breast for not much more than a few bucks per pound.

Let's start by reminding ourselves what goes into getting meat into grocery stores. First, you feed a cow twenty to thirty pounds of grain—typically alfalfa, soy, and corn—per day. You give her lots of water—as much as 20 gallons per day. Remember, 2.2 pounds of beef requires 55 pounds of food and almost 4,000 gallons of water. Raising and slaughtering some seventy billion land animals each year worldwide requires so many resources that more than a quarter of the earth's terrestrial surface is used for livestock grazing, while a third of all arable land is used by livestock feed crop cultivation, according to the United Nations Food and Agriculture Organization.[100] And yet meat is very cheap. How is such an inefficient source of food so affordable for consumers?

Quite simply, because of you.

First there's the marketing dollars. Remember "Beef. It's What's for Dinner," "Pork. The Other White Meat," and "Got Milk?" These massive marketing campaigns were spearheaded by the federal government during the '90s to get more people to eat meat, dairy, and eggs. Thanks to Congress, the industry is actually required to set aside a portion of their sales into so-called checkoff programs, which are used to research and market those products. If the government forced e-cigarette companies to run vaping ads on TV targeted toward kids, the public would be outraged. Why aren't we outraged that our elected representatives are rubberstamping more than $500 million worth of advertisements for products that are just as addicting and unhealthy as smoking?

**Taxpayers are subsidizing these foods to the tune of $38 billion per year.**

That's only the start. Not only do government-mandated ads compel people to buy more meat, dairy, and eggs, taxpayers are subsidizing these foods to the tune of $38 billion per year. You probably don't even notice that every five to seven years Congress passes a "Farm Bill." It barely makes the news, since it's one of the few things Republicans and Democrats tend to agree on. (The 2018 farm bill passed 386–47 in the House and 87–13 in the Senate.[101]) How bad could something with such a bland name be?

Very bad. While parts of the bill are important, such as funding food stamps for struggling

Americans, most of it amounts to a windfall for billion-dollar agriculture companies. The original farm bills were passed during the Great Depression to help struggling farmers by authorizing the government to purchase excess supplies of crops. It's a different story nowadays. Between 1995 and 2009, taxpayers doled out more than $160 billion in subsidies, but two-thirds of American farmers received nothing. "The funds mostly went to big corporate players, with one-fifth of recipients grabbing nine-tenths of the cash,"[102] explains lawyer David Simon in his book *Meatonomics*.

And where does most of that money go? Growing cheap crops meant solely for farm animals. In fact, of the three hundred million acres of food planted in the United States, half are corn and soy.[103] Fruits and vegetables meant for humans are grown on a mere fourteen million acres. All together, Simon calculates that ranchers sell their cows for as much as $90 less than they would cost to rear without taxpayer subsidies, while pigs sell for $8 less.[104] If the subsidies were to go away, meat and dairy would cost a lot more, and consumers would buy a lot less.

It gets worse. In 2019, NPR reported that the United States was sitting on a 1.4 billion–pound cheese surplus: "The glut, which at 900,000 cubic yards is the largest in US history, means that there is enough cheese sitting in cold storage to wrap around the US Capitol."[105] Even though Americans are consuming less cheese and drinking less milk than they used to, taxpayer subsidies continue to incentivize dairy companies to pump out as much product as possible.

Yes, the federal government publicly recommends that half your plate be filled with fruits and vegetables, but it's quietly making sure that it's instead packed with beef, chicken, eggs, and processed junk food. Or, as Ferd Hoefner, the former policy director for the National Sustainable Agriculture Coalition, explained, "We've locked up food production with a policy that says, 'Thou shalt not grow fruits and vegetables.'"[106]

**FOLLOW THE MONEY:**

Between 1995 and 2009, taxpayers doled out more than $160 billion in subsidies, but two-thirds of American farmers received nothing.

# PANDEMICS LIKE COVID-19 ARE PREVENTABLE

Here's a word you probably don't know but should (and one you'll be hearing more about): *zoonotic*. Although it sounds like being hypnotized by a zoo, it refers to illnesses that are caused by viruses, bacteria, or parasites transmitted between animals and humans, and then from person to person—which is, for example, exactly how the coronavirus pandemic began.

According to the US Centers for Disease Control and Prevention, about 60 percent of all known infectious diseases and 73 percent of emerging ones are of zoonotic origin. This can happen when people come into contact with the flesh or bodily fluids of sick animals, whether they're domestic livestock or wild creatures hunted for food.

As humans press ever farther into wildlife habitats and travel and trade globally, these potentially deadly germs are more frequently spread around the world with us. And industrial-scale factory farming only aggravates the problem. Each year, tens of thousands of Americans fall ill from animal-borne illnesses, especially babies, the elderly, and those with compromised immune systems. A 2012 report by the International Livestock Research Institute found that animal-to-human diseases kill more than two million people each year, mostly in low- to middle-income countries, and that most of those infections come from livestock.

Here's how some of the headline-making outbreaks have been linked to carnivory:

- **COVID-19:** It will take the world countless years to recover from the devastating effects of this pandemic. Experts widely agree that COVID-19, which is caused by the coronavirus SARS-CoV-2, originated in a "wet" market—a large marketplace that sells fresh meat, fish, and produce. With thousands of people and live and slaughtered animals packed closely together, novel viruses can spawn and spread easily, which is precisely what happened in Wuhan, China, near the end of 2019.

- **Bird flu (aka avian influenza):** The causal virus is found naturally in wild waterbirds, but it can infect domestic chickens and other poultry and then spread to humans via their blood or undercooked meat. Avian influenza germs sometimes combine with similar human flu strains to create dangerous epidemics like the Spanish flu of 1918–1919, which afflicted half a billion people worldwide.

- **Swine flu:** This airborne, virus-caused respiratory disease causes regular outbreaks in pigs, and pork farmers (and some pork-eaters) are more likely than others to get it from the infected swine. As with bird flu, the human and porcine versions of the virus can combine and spread further.

- **Ebola:** This often deadly, highly contagious disease, marked by severe pain, diarrhea, and internal bleeding, is spread by contact with bodily fluids from infected people. The 2014 outbreak (which the World Health Organization estimated to have killed at least 5,000 people) emerged from Central Africa and is believed to have been contracted by individuals who had handled or eaten infected bushmeat. Unprocessed wild animal meats—including nonhuman primates, antelope, and bats, among others—are a major source of protein for rural people near tropical forests in parts of the developing world, so it's an ongoing risk.

- **AIDS (Acquired Immunodeficiency Syndrome):** This disease is caused by a virus called HIV, and is also linked to bushmeat, most likely an infected chimpanzee in West Africa. Although AIDS became prominent in the news in the early 1980s, scientists now believe it probably emerged decades earlier. According to the AIDS Institute, the simian version of HIV most likely mutated into the human version after people who hunted the animals for food encountered the monkeys' infected blood.

A simple summary: We have outgrown the dated system of using animals to produce meat and milk. It's killing us in too many ways.

# YOU WILL HAVE
# SERIOUSLY
# GOOD POOPS

We've already talked about the problems of animal poop (see page 79). Now, let's talk about yours. Did you know that, according to the National Institute of Diabetes and Digestive and Kidney Diseases (NIDDK), about 16 percent of adults have symptoms of constipation, as do about 33 percent of adults over sixty? Now, did you know how rare constipation is among vegans? Although there haven't been enough rigorous studies to be sure, go ahead and ask vegans about their bowel movements (always a fun topic at dinner) and you will almost inevitably get the same answer: "Ever since I've been vegan, I poop *all the time!*"

That's because fiber, which is found only in plant food (see page 21), adds bulk to stool, which keeps things moving through your intestines. According to a 2016 study published in the journal *Clinical Nutrition Research*, people who followed a nonmeat diet loaded with fruits and vegetables for twelve weeks reported less constipation.[107] This is partly because meat takes as long as four days to move through your body (during which time it begins to rot), while plants typically pass through within twenty-four hours.

The American Dietetic Association recommends that people eat about 20 to 35 grams of fiber daily. How much does the average American consume? About 5 to 15 grams. All told, 95 percent of Americans are fiber-deficient, with most adults and teens barely eating half the recommended amount.[108] Meanwhile, someone who eats a whole-food, plant-based diet wolfs down around 41 grams of wonderful, poop-enhancing fiber each day.[109]

Eat fiber. Your bowels will thank you.

**FIBER FACT:** In 2018, Americans spent about $1.43 billion on laxatives. Think how much broccoli and spinach that could buy.[110]

# DOGS AND CATS AREN'T THE ONLY LOVING ANIMALS

Did you know that some countries raise and slaughter dogs for dinner? Though it's quite common in some cultures, it may be horrifying to think that an animal you consider to be a faithful companion could suffer the fate of a food animal. In the United States, we are told from a young age that cows and chickens are brought into this world to be food; dogs and cats are not.

But, when you think about it, why does the thought of eating a cow make our mouths water, but the thought of eating a dog make us want to throw up? What is the difference, truly, between your family dog who sleeps at the foot of your bed and the cow who ends up on a dinner plate? Is one less emotional than the other? Is one cuter, more entertaining? Does one deserve to live in peace while the other is led down a dark, noisy tunnel to slaughter? It's all really just a matter of how we're socialized to believe it's okay to eat one animal but not the other. As Dr. Melanie Joy, author of *Why We Love Dogs, Eat Pigs and Wear Cows*, says, "We send one species to the butcher and give our love and kindness to another apparently for no reason other than because *it's the way things are*. When our attitudes and behaviors toward animals are so inconsistent, and this inconsistency is so unexamined, we can safely say we have been fed absurdities. It is absurd that we eat pigs and love dogs and don't even know why. Many of us spend long minutes in the aisle of the drugstore mulling over what toothpaste to buy. Yet most of us don't spend any time at all thinking about what species of animal we eat and why. Our choices as consumers drive an industry that kills ten billion animals per year in the United States alone."[111]

All animals feel. They love. They trust. They fear. They connect. They worry. They grieve. They look for comfort. They have unique and interesting personalities. They don't want to die. They do everything they can to avoid pain. Every last one of them, whether dog or cat or cow or chicken or goat or lamb or human. Every last one of them is capable of joy and pain. Some of us are smarter than others, some larger, some more fierce, some more neurotic and needy.

A good thought experiment is to just think for a minute before you eat an animal food: Does my taste for this dish override what happened to this one animal on my plate? Am I at peace with what she or he went through?

# IT'S BASIC:
# DO UNTO OTHERS

If you wouldn't want to be shot up with chemicals and growth hormones from the second you were born, forced to spend your entire brief life in filth where you could hardly breathe, become so fat and in so much pain that you could barely move, heaved to slaughter amid the terrified sounds of peers—all before you were barely an adolescent— and, finally, lie dead on someone's dinner plate, picked over by some distracted person who takes a few bites of your seasoned flesh before scraping the rest into the trash can because he's not in the mood for your flavor after all . . . well then, you might not want to eat meat, dairy, or eggs.

Why? Because karma might just be a thing: What you put out into the world eventually comes back around to you. It's a very simple idea: Treat others—human and animal—as you would like to be treated.

If you don't care about what happened to the animal before it arrived on your plate, you're helping to create a world that might not care so much about you. Kindness begets kindness. Cruelty begets cruelty. Being awake and aware and choosing consciously what you eat means you help to create a world that is more awake and aware, a world where conscious choices have made it a better place to live.

The alternative is pretty bleak.

# WILDLIFE IS KILLED
# TO PROTECT ANIMAL
# AGRICULTURE

We seriously wish this were a tinfoil-hat conspiracy theory. But there actually is a little-known branch of the United States Department of Agriculture dedicated to killing wild animals—many of them endangered—just to protect other animals that are raised to become food.

Wildlife Services (a bit of an oxymoron considering what they do) spends millions of our tax dollars every year setting leg traps and neck snares, spreading poison, dispatching hired guns in helicopters, and training dogs to tear apart whatever wildlife might be deemed a threat to livestock. Raccoons, beavers, great horned owls, eagles, coyotes, bears, foxes, and countless other creatures get caught in the traps and die slow, agonizing deaths.

**The traps are set for wild animals, but they snare neighboring dogs and cats, too.**

In 2016 alone, Wildlife Services admitted to killing over 1.5 million native animals nationwide, animals who were simply going about their lives grazing, hunting, and wandering as wild animals do.[112] This is how it happens, as PETA explains: The animal—a coyote or bear or raccoon, for example—"steps on the steel-jaw trap spring, the trap's jaws slam shut, clamping down on the animal's limb or paw. As the animal struggles in excruciating pain to get free, the steel vise cuts into his or her flesh—often down to the bone—mutilating the leg or paw. Some animals, especially mothers desperate to return to their young, will even attempt to chew or twist off their trapped limbs. Animals often struggle for hours, sometimes days, before they finally succumb to exhaustion, exposure, frostbite, shock, and death."[113] The traps are set for wild animals, but they snare neighboring dogs and cats, too.

So here we have an army of trappers and aerial shooters using our tax dollars to exterminate millions of wild animals every year in order to protect a rancher's revenue-generating cows and lambs—so that those same cows and lambs can then be slaughtered for meat: a high price to pay for a burger.

# **66**

# **YOU COULD WARD OFF ALZHEIMER'S**

Heart disease might be America's No. 1 killer (and almost completely preventable), but Alzheimer's disease and other forms of dementia are quickly becoming the most difficult and emotionally painful conditions to manage. Alzheimer's is known as "the long goodbye" for a good reason: Whereas a heart attack can kill us in an instant, Alzheimer's takes years. In the process, it robs us of our faculties, eroding cherished memories and destroying our ability to be independent. It places enormous burdens not just on victims, but family members who must witness their loved ones slowly fading away while requiring ever more care. Tending to dementia patients is also placing extreme stress on our healthcare system, costing some $290 billion per year according to the Alzheimer's Association. This figure will only continue to skyrocket, with a projected 7.1 million seniors expected to suffer from dementia by 2025, an increase of nearly 30 percent compared with 2019.

The science of Alzheimer's disease is still not clear. Despite billions of dollars' worth of research, there remains no effective treatment. Fortunately, there is compelling science suggesting that we might be able to prevent it from developing—and for adults with mild cognitive impairment, prevent it from escalating to full-blown dementia.

You guessed it: The answer is plants. Neurologists Ayesha Sherzai, MD, and Dean Sherzai, MD, PhD, are a husband-and-wife duo at the forefront of Alzheimer's research. While most funding is devoted to medication that can manage symptoms of the disease, the Sherzais, who are directors of the Alzheimer's Prevention Program at Loma Linda Medical Center, are part of a small group of pioneers who want to prevent it altogether. After years of studying the disease and analyzing studies involving hundreds of thousands of people, they have come across a startling, if controversial, conclusion: Alzheimer's disease is chiefly a lifestyle disease, not a genetic one. In fact, they say, 90 percent of us can avoid Alzheimer's entirely if we eat the right foods.

> **You guessed it: The answer is plants.**

"The best diet for brain health is full of whole foods like greens, legumes, berries, and whole grains, and is very low in animal fats, saturated fats, and salt,"[114] they explain. In conjunction with regular exercise, good sleep, stress management, and cognitive games that challenge the brain's capacities, we can keep our brains sharp well into our twilight years.

According to the Drs. Sherzai, Alzheimer's is "essentially a garbage disposal problem" caused by the brain's "inability to cope with what we feed it over a lifetime."[115] And what is this "garbage"? Meat, dairy, eggs, and processed foods. Each of these foods cause inflammation and the buildup of oxidative by-products that clog blood vessels and deprive your noggin of vital oxygen and nutrients. And while the vast majority of Alzheimer's patients are senior citizens, the disease begins to take form decades earlier. That's why it's never too early to start eating brain-healthy food.

But it's also never too late: "Our combined research is revealing that early signs of cognitive decline can be reversed,"[116] the Sherzais explain.

So, whether you're turning eighteen or eighty, remember to keep fruits, vegetables, and whole grains on the brain.

## A STARTLING, IF CONTROVERSIAL, CONCLUSION:

Alzheimer's disease is chiefly a lifestyle disease, not a genetic one.

# GOING VEGAN

## HELPS PREVENT AND

## TREAT ARTHRITIS

A re you one of the 350 million adults who suffer from arthritis across the globe? If not, you certainly know someone who does. In the United States, arthritis is the leading cause of disability among seniors; it can even affect the young: Three hundred thousand babies and kids suffer from arthritis in America, according to the CDC.

Arthritis is a general term that describes more than a hundred types of joint diseases, typically presenting as inflammation and stiffness. In simple terms, the painful swelling occurs when the lining of your joints, known as the synovium, swells due to an increase of synovial fluid. As blood and synovial fluid flood the joint, it swells and causes an excess of inflammatory proteins that are pushed into nearby soft tissue. The result is pain in and around the joints of your body, commonly in the hands, wrists, elbows, shoulders, knees, ankles, feet, jaw, and neck. Arthritis can be a crippling condition that saps older adults of their mobility and independence.

But in many cases it can be prevented. And if you have it, you can drastically decrease your discomfort.

The key is that big *I* word: inflammation. It's the root of so many health issues, from heart disease to cancer, and arthritis is no exception. If you don't believe us, take it from the Arthritis Foundation, which might know a thing or two about arthritis. They concluded, after studying fifty-three arthritic patients in a controlled setting, that "diets that include animal products (e.g., dairy, red meat) exacerbate the [patients'] symptoms likely due to their pro-inflammatory effects. In contrast, diets rich in vegetables, fruits, and fiber are associated with lower BMI, have anti-inflammatory properties, and help reduce pain and inflammation."[117]

There's more: A 2015 study of about forty people with arthritis found that those who eat a whole-food, plant-based diet can significantly reduce pain due to osteoarthritis in just two weeks.[118] According to the Physicians Committee for Responsible Medicine (PCRM): "By the end of the six-week study, [the patients] reported more energy and better physical functioning, too." As we know, plants are high in fiber, which, in addition to making your poops smoother, also smooths out your joints. According to a study published in the *Annals of the Rheumatic Diseases*, people who consume the highest amount of dietary fiber had as much as a 61 percent lower risk of knee arthritis.[119]

**"Diets rich in vegetables, fruits, and fiber help reduce pain and inflammation."**

In case you were wondering, here are the foods that exacerbate inflammation and arthritic pain: red meat, sugar, fat, salt, and dairy.[120]

# VEGAN IS SEXY

As you read earlier, men on vegan diets have harder and longer-lasting erections (see page 28). Women have more blood flowing through their tender bits so they get more lubricated and turned on (see page 29). Thus, in purely physical terms, eating vegan sets you up for the sexual equipment to work well. But unclogging the fatty deposits (from meat and dairy) that larded up your arteries isn't just good for circulation.

Sexual attraction begins in the brain, so the better you feel about yourself, the more open you'll likely be to your partner . . . especially if they are also on the path with you. There's nothing sexier than someone who has curiosity, an open heart, and a willingness to grow and change with you. That conscious combo is the stuff of bliss. When a person understands that our vulnerable animal friends need protecting rather than exploiting, that's hot. We are sexiest when we are both tender and bold: A tender heart recognizes the plight of animals, and a bold person takes initiative to stop eating them.

Lastly and most importantly, when both partners eat vegan, you have a bond built on shared values, and that makes sex an expression of something deep and foundational—which is seriously sexy.

# #CHOCOLATE

Great news, everyone: Chocolate is essentially cocoa, cocoa butter (which is basically just the vegetable fat extracted from the cocoa bean), sugar, and a few (ideally zero) additives, such as lecithin or vanilla—and all these are vegan.

However, not all chocolate is plant-based, including milk chocolate, although some manufacturers are creating plant-based milk chocolates from almond or other nondairy milks. And just because the label says "dark" chocolate doesn't mean it's dairy-free; ingredients that are derived from milk may still be present, such as whey, casein, or milk fat. Best to stick to chocolate with a cocoa content of 70 percent or more.

If you're jonesing for more than just a chocolate bar, there are more excellent vegan desserts to choose from than you could ever eat. We always ask Fran Costigan, Queen of Vegan Desserts, for her recipes. Here is one of our favorites.

# Fran's Chocolate Peanut Butter Spread

*A three-ingredient chocolate peanut butter spread to use on everything. Eating off a spoon counts, too! (Can be made with other nut spreads.)*

½ cup chocolate chips (3 ounces)

5 tablespoons of your favorite plant milk (anything but rice or hemp)

3 tablespoons peanut butter, smooth or crunchy, more to taste

**1** Put the chocolate chips into a microwavable jar. Pour the plant milk over the chips.

Microwave on high power for 20 seconds. Check to see if the chocolate has started to melt, then microwave on high power again for 15 seconds.

**2** Stir until the chocolate has melted and you have made a nice smooth chocolate spread.

If the chocolate is not fully melted, microwave again, just for a few seconds. Stir in the peanut butter.

Great with toast, greater with toast and jam, and even greater with jam and sliced bananas.

**MAKES ½ CUP**

# ANIMAL PRODUCTS
# ARE LINKED
# TO CANCER

While there's no magic bullet when it comes to cancer, research suggests that whole plant foods like vegetables, fruits, whole grains, and beans are protective. Animal products are not.

It isn't just that animal foods lack health-promoting fiber and phytochemicals; they contain substances that encourage cancer cells to spread exponentially. Here are five ways animal foods contribute to cancer risk, brought to you by Lee Crosby, RD, LD, registered dietitian with the Barnard Medical Center:

1   **Saturated fat:** Animal foods are often high in saturated fat, which has been linked to increased risk of breast cancer, ovarian cancer, aggressive prostate cancer, and even lung cancer. What's the connection? For one thing, consuming lots of saturated fat can make the body less sensitive to insulin, the hormone that lowers blood sugar. To overcome this insulin resistance, the body pumps out more insulin even as blood sugar rises—a dangerous combination that can trigger cancer cells to grow. (And even a lot of fish

and so-called lean meat like chicken breast are loaded with saturated fat.)

2  **Heterocyclic Amines (HCAs) and Polycyclic Aromatic Hydrocarbons (PAHs):** HCAs and PAHs are cancer-causing baddies that form when animal flesh—including beef, pork, chicken, and fish—are cooked at high temperatures. Think frying, pan-frying, and grilling. HCAs form on the surface of flesh foods when creatine or creatinine found in meat reacts with protein. PAHs, on the other hand, result when fat drips from meat onto a hot surface or fire. The resulting carcinogenic smoke coats the meat with these tiny cancer bombs.

3  **N-Nitroso Compounds (NOCs):** Many processed meats, like deli meats, bacon, sausage, and ham, are preserved with nitrates and nitrites. These chemicals help prevent the growth of deadly botulism bacteria and give these products an attractive pink color. Not so attractive: colorectal cancer caused by the NOCs that form when those chemicals react with substances in the meat during cooking and digestion. But fresh red meat isn't off the hook—when we digest red meat, we form these hazardous NOCs in our intestines.

4  **Persistent Organic Pollutants (POPs):** POPs are toxic chemicals found nearly everywhere in the environment. They're usually by-products of pesticide use and industrial processes, and are found in wind,

water, soil, and even plants! However, they tend to build up in animal fat. When humans eat animals or drink their milk, they are exposed to a hefty dose of POPs. Interestingly, "healthy" fatty fish are some of the worst culprits. Beyond their links to cancer, POPs can also interfere with fertility and may even increase the risk of diabetes.

5   **IGF-1:** Insulinlike growth factor, or IGF-1, is a substance made by the body that tells cancer cells to grow, baby, grow. People who eat adequate protein from plants (about 10 percent of their calories) have been found to have lower levels of IGF-1 than those eating diets higher in protein from mostly meat and dairy products. So, best to stick to whole plant foods for healthy IGF-1 levels.

## THE CANCER CELL CHEER SQUAD:

It isn't just that animal foods lack health-promoting fiber and phytochemicals; they contain substances that encourage cancer cells to spread exponentially.

# FISH FEEL PAIN

Who doesn't like *Finding Nemo*? Nemo is funny—the whole movie is—partly because everyone's favorite little fish has plenty of amazing adventures without being hooked, filleted, and turned into a meal instead of a movie—a plight shared by trillions (yes, trillions) of fish each year.

"Okay," your Uncle Albert says, "but fish don't really feel pain. I'll give you cows and sheep, maybe. But fish? They don't seem to mind it when I catch them with my rod and reel. I've never heard a fish even cry out."

True, fish don't moan and groan. But they do feel pain. In her meticulously researched book, *Do Fish Feel Pain?*, biologist Victoria Braithwaite concludes from her many years of studies that fish may suffer from pain just as much as birds and mammals.

What makes an animal feel pain is its nervous system, and fish have well-developed systems with the same kind of analgesic hormones, such as endorphins, that humans have and rely on to process pain. Lynne Sneddon, director of bioveterinary science at the University of Liverpool, was the first scientist to discover that fish possess the nerves—the same nerve types that detect painful stimuli in humans—known as pain receptors. Sneddon showed that pinching and pricking fish activates these nerve fibers, explaining: "My research has shown that fish have a strikingly similar neuronal system to mammals."[121]

Moreover, according to Dr. Culum Brown of Australia's Macquarie University, the stress that fish experience when they're caught on a hook and thrown on a boat might exceed the stress that humans feels when they drown. "Unlike drowning in humans, where we die in about 4 to 5 minutes because we can't extract any oxygen from water, fish can go on for much longer," he explains. "It's a prolonged slow death most of the time, which is pretty horrible, when you think about it."[122]

Fish are also a great deal smarter than humans previously thought. Depending on the species, they possess excellent long-term memories, can cooperate with one another in skills and tasks, and have figured out how to use tools to achieve goals. They can recognize each other (guppies can identify up to fifteen other guppies . . . and they totally prefer hanging out with their BFFs). And they also exhibit social learning (they pass knowledge about their environment on to their fellow fish). In the early 2000s researchers at the Red Sea witnessed groupers and morays hunting cooperatively; after one

> **"Fish have a strikingly similar neuronal system to mammals."**

grouper chased a fish into a crevice, the grouper swam fifteen meters to a cave, fetched a moray back to the hiding prey, and then used posture to indicate the hiding fish. Previously, only ravens, chimpanzees, and humans were known to use what is called "referential gesturing." It indicates that a grouper knows that a moray, too, can know: That, in turn, is called "theory of mind," and means that fish have a lot more going on inside their brains than anyone ever thought.[123]

Additionally, according to research published in *Royal Society Open Science*, fish exhibit behaviors and brain chemistry almost identical to those of very stressed and depressed people—behaviors particularly noticeable in horribly overcrowded fish farms. Up to a quarter of fish in fish farms have stunted growth and float lifelessly at the surface of the tanks. Some scientists have likened the behavior of these fish, known as "drop outs," to suicide.

All this is why SmithsonianMag.com published an article in January 2018 titled "It's Official: Fish Feel Pain." So, although only a fish could tell you if the pain he feels is similar to the pain you would feel if someone hooked your mouth and threw you into the ocean, it's still pain. It still hurts.[‡]

‡ By the way, if you think that throwing the fish back after catching it gets you (and him) off the hook, think again. Even fish who are thrown back may soon die: Hooks, exhaustion, and sometimes excessive pressure when the fish is brought to the surface can all contribute to loss of life. Just the mere trauma of capture, even for short periods, can herald death.

# THIS LIFESTYLE
# IS AN ONGOING
# ADVENTURE

Y ou can take this as far as you want: After
going animal-free in your diet, and having
had a chance to enjoy your enhanced health
and uplifted soul, you might want to think about
moving away from wearing leather, fur, and down.
Even wool.

Veganism is best taken on, in our humble
opinion, gradually and in the spirit of exploration.
Rather than feeling deprived, like "Oh my God, it's
one more thing I have to give up," we prefer the
attitude of, "Oh wow, there are so many amazing
alternatives to animal products. I'm all over this!" It
becomes an adventure finding all kinds of new and
stylish products, from faux leather shoes to super
soft comforters made without feathers. Cosmetics,
too, tend to be purer and kinder to the skin when
they are made without animal ingredients.

We're not hardcore absolutists. If you like tot-
ing that leather handbag, that's your business, not
ours. Proud of your best wool suit? Wear it. But
when it's time to replace these articles, think about
animal-free alternatives. Do what you can and keep
moving forward. As much as you might be enjoying
this newfound way of eating, we recommend you
take the next right step that calls to you.

# Acknowledgments

### KATHY

Big love and gratitude goes to Dan Buettner for sharing his wisdom on the Blue Zones over margaritas and thick bean soups. A deep bow to Jennifer Barrett, who invited me (and thus you!) into her farm to see the truth about raising animals for food. Huge thanks to Lee Crosby, RD, LD, for making so clear why diet and cancer are linked. So much appreciation to Noam Mohr for his incredibly well-researched work on statistics about eating animals. A shout-out to Dotsie Bausch and Switch4Good for the great dairy info and graphic. And thanks to Tal Ronnen for gifting the world with cashew cream.

### GENE

Thank you Miranda Spencer, for all the editorial help you always provide. And Chris Hays, for your constant care and support.

### BOTH OF US

Thanks to all the people at Workman who did such a great job helping us make this book: Our wonderful editor, Megan Nicolay; our publisher (and friend), Suzie Bolotin; and the rest of the team: Rae Ann Spitzenberger, Dylan Julian, Sarah Curley, Ciara Patten, Barbara Peragine, Doug Wolff, and

Chloe Puton. And most of all, we are grateful to Nick Bromley, without whose humor, intelligence, and editorial genius this book could not and would not have happened. Thanks, Nick!

And to you, our dear readers, we are so very grateful you were called to this book. Keep in touch and let us know how you're doing. Join us on social media (@genestone2022 and @kathyfreston), and use the hashtag #ReasonsToBeVegan so we can keep the conversation going. We'll see you out there!

# Notes

**1** Janet Forgrieve, "The Growing Acceptance of Veganism," *Forbes*, November 2, 2018, https://www.forbes.com/sites/janetforgrieve /2018/11/02/picturing-a-kindler-gentler-world-vegan-month /#353308032f2b.

**2** "Vegan Burgers Outselling Meat in Healthy Fast Food Chain LEON," *Vegconomist*, published January 28, 2020, https://vegconomist.com /food-and-beverage/vegan-burgers-outselling-meat-in-healthy-fast-food -chain-leon/.

**3** University of Adelaide, "Study Shows Potential for Reduced Methane from Cows," Phys.org, July 5, 2019, https://phys.org /news/2019-07-potential-methane-cows.html.

**4** Brian Merchant, "Charbroiling a Burger Pollutes More Than Driving an 18-Wheeler 143 Miles," *Vice*, September 22, 2012, https://www.vice.com/en_us/article/jppvdy/charbroiling-a-burger -pollutes-more-than-driving-an-18-wheeler-143-miles.

**5** Rina Raphael, "Meatless Burgers vs. Beef: How Beyond Meat's Environmental Impact Stacks Up," *Fast Company*, September 26, 2018, https://www.fastcompany.com/90241836/meatless-burgers-vs-beef -how-beyond-meats-environmental-impact-stacks-up.

**6** "Soy and Health," Physicians Committee for Responsible Medicine, accessed July 12, 2019, https://www.pcrm.org/good-nutrition /nutrition-information/soy-and-health.

**7** "Soy and Breast Cancer," The Academy of Nutrition and Dietetics, accessed July 12, 2019, https://www.oncologynutrition.org/erfc /healthy-nutrition-now/foods/soy-and-breast-cancer.

**8** Todd Nippoldt, "Is It True That People Who Have Hypothyroidism Should Avoid Soy?" Mayo Clinic, accessed July 13, 2019, https://www.mayoclinic.org/diseases-conditions/hypothyroidism /expert-answers/hyperthyroidism/faq-20058188.

**9** Dave Carter, "Dairy Cows Produce 61% More Milk Than 25 Years Ago," New Hope Network, August 28, 2012, https://www.newhope .com/blog/dairy-cows-produce-61-more-milk-25-years-ago.

**10** Michael Greger, "How Much Pus Is There in Milk?" NutritionFacts .org, September 8, 2011, https://nutritionfacts.org/2011/09/08 /how-much-pus-is-there-in-milk/.

**11** Alicja Kucharska, et al., "Significance of Diet in Treated and Untreated Acne Vulgaris," *Advances in Dermatology and Allergology* 33, no. 2 (April 2016): 81–86.

**12** Clement Adebamowo, et al., "Milk Consumption and Acne in Adolescent Girls," *Dermatology Online Journal* 12, no. 4 (May 2006): 1.

**13** "Lactose Intolerance," US National Library of Medicine, accessed September 5, 2019, https://ghr.nlm.nih.gov/condition/lactose-intolerance#statistics.

**14** John Ross, "Bad Bug, No Drugs: The Real End of Antibiotics?" Harvard Medical School, February 27, 2017, https://www.health.harvard.edu/blog/bad-bug-no-drugs-real-end-antibiotics-2017022711103.

**15** C. Lee Ventola, "The Antibiotic Resistance Crisis," *Pharmacy and Therapeutics* 40, no. 4 (April 2015): 277–83.

**16** Chris Dall, "FDA: Antibiotic Use in Food Animals Continues to Rise," Center for Infectious Disease Research and Policy, December 22, 2016, http://www.cidrap.umn.edu/news-perspective/2016/12/fda-antibiotic-use-food-animals-continues-rise.

**17** "Heart Disease & Erectile Dysfunction," The Cleveland Clinic, accessed May 25, 2020, https://my.clevelandclinic.org/health/diseases/15029-heart-disease—erectile-dysfunction.

**18** "How High Blood Pressure Leads to Erectile Dysfunction," WebMD, accessed May 25, 2020, https://www.webmd.com/hypertension-high-blood-pressure/guide/high-blood-pressure-erectile-dysfunction#1.

**19** "EPA Study Reveals Contamination of Fish in U.S. Lakes and Reservoirs," *The Lincoln Journal Star*, November 10, 2009, https://journalstar.com/news/state-and-regional/nebraska/epa-study-reveals-contamination-of-fish-in-u-s-lakes/article_188c6a38-ce46-11de-9f4d-001cc4c03286.html.

**20** "Study Finds Toxic Pollutants in Fish Across the World's Oceans," Scripps Institution of Oceanography (press release), January 28, 2016, https://scripps.ucsd.edu/news/study-finds-toxic-pollutants-fish-across-worlds-oceans.

**21** M. Berners Lee, et al., "Current Global Food Production Is Sufficient to Meet Human Nutritional Needs in 2050 Provided There Is Radical Societal Adaptation," *Elementa: Science of the Anthropocene* 6, no. 1 (July 2018): 52.

**22** Joanne Slavin and Justin Carlson, "Carbohydrates," *Advances in Nutrition* 5, no. 6 (November 2014): 760–61.

**23** Sara Seidelmann, et al., "Dietary Carbohydrate Intake and Mortality: A Prospective Cohort Study and Meta-Analysis," *The Lancet Public Health* 3, no. 9 (September 1, 2018): e419–e428.

**24** Heli Virtanen, et al., "Intake of Different Dietary Proteins and Risk of Heart Failure in Men," *Circulation: Heart Failure* 11, no. 6 (published online May 29, 2018).

**25** "Are Humans Supposed to Eat Meat?" peta2, May 28, 2015, https://www.peta2.com/news/humans-supposed-eat-meat/.

**26** Marla Paul, "Eating Eggs and Cholesterol Linked to Heart Disease and Death Risk," Northwestern Medicine, March 15, 2019, https://news.feinberg.northwestern.edu/2019/03/eating-eggs-and-cholesterol-linked-to-heart-disease-and-death-risk/.

**27** Jamie Ducharme, "Eggs May Be Bad for the Heart, a New Study Says—But There's More to the Story," *Time*, March 15, 2019, https://time.com/5551508/are-eggs-bad-for-you/.

**28** Michael Greger, "Eggs & Breast Cancer," NutritionFacts.org, January 14, 2019, https://nutritionfacts.org/video/eggs-and-breast-cancer/.

**29** Ibid.

**30** E. L. Richman, S. A. Kenfield, M. J. Stampfer, E. L. Giovannucci, and J. M. Chan, "Egg, Red Meat, and Poultry Intake and Risk of Lethal Prostate Cancer in the Prostate-Specific Antigen-Era: Incidence and Survival," *Cancer Prevention Research* 4, no. 12 (published ahead of print; September 2011), https://doi.org/10.1158/1940-6207.CAPR-11-0354.

**31** Chris Crowley, "A New Warning Says We Could Run Out of Fish by 2048," *HuffPost*, updated December 14, 2017, https://www.huffpost.com/entry/a-new-warning-says-we-cou_b_13615338.

**32** Azua Zizhan Luo, "Ocean Fish Stocks on 'Verge of Collapse,' Says IRIN Report," *New Security Beat* (blog), February 28, 2017, https://www.newsecuritybeat.org/2017/02/ocean-fish-stocks-on-verge-collapse-irin-report/.

**33** "Bycatch—A Sad Topic," The Fish Forward Project, accessed July 23, 2019, https://www.fishforward.eu/en/project/by-catch/.

**34** "Overfishing," The World Wildlife Fund, accessed July 24, 2019, https://www.worldwildlife.org/threats/overfishing.

**35** Fred Pearce, "No More Seafood by 2050?" *New Scientist*, November 2, 2006, https://www.newscientist.com/article/dn10433-no-more-seafood-by-2050/.

**36** "PCBs in Farmed Salmon," The Environmental Working Group, July 31, 2003, https://www.ewg.org/research/pcbs-farmed-salmon.

**37** "Rain Forest Threats," *National Geographic*, accessed August 12, 2019, https://www.nationalgeographic.com/environment/habitats/rainforest-threats/.

**38** "Cattle Ranching in the Amazon Region," Yale School of Forestry & Environmental Studies, accessed October 14, 2019, https://globalforestatlas.yale.edu/amazon/land-use/cattle-ranching.

**39** Geoff Watts, "The Cows That Could Help Fight Climate Change," BBC, August 6, 2019, https://www.bbc.com/future/article/20190806 -how-vaccines-could-fix-our-problem-with-cow-emissions.

**40** Ursula Perano, "Brazil Has Lost 1,330 Square Miles of Amazon Rainforest Under Bolsonaro," *Axios*, July 28, 2019, https://www .axios.com/amazon-rainforest-bolsonaro-brazil-south-america -fda08c12-0de2-43ce-93f0-d02709b18e7b.html.

**41** "Meat's Large Water Footprint: Why Raising Livestock and Poultry for Meat is so Resource-Intensive," Foodtank, accessed October 1, 2019, https://foodtank.com/news/2013/12/why-meat-eats-resources/.

**42** Jonathan Parks-Ramage, "1,800 Gallons of Water Goes Into One Pound of Meat," *Vice*, June 2, 2017, https://www.vice.com/en_us /article/d3z8az/1800-gallons-of-water-goes-into-one-pound-of-meat.

**43** "The United States Meat Industry at a Glance," North American Meat Institute, accessed May 25, 2020, https://www.meatinstitute .org/index.php?ht=d/sp/i/47465/pid/47465.

**44** Rachel Curit, "How Does Eating Meat Impact Your Water Footprint?" One Green Planet, accessed May 25, 2020, https://www.onegreen planet.org/animalsandnature/how-does-eating-meat-impact-your -water-footprint/.

**45** Joe McCarthy, "Over Half the World Could Face Water Shortage by 2050," Global Citizen, March 19, 2018, https://www.global citizen.org/en/content/water-shortages-un-report-2050-climate-change/.

**46** Gene Stone (ed.), *Forks Over Knives: The Plant-Based Way to Health* (New York: The Experiment, 2011), 40.

**47** "Dehorning: Dairy's Dark Secret," PETA, accessed June 30, 2019, https://www.peta.org/issues/animals-used-for-food/factory-farming /cows/dairy-industry/dehorning/.

**48** "What's Wrong with Wearing Wool?" PETA, accessed July 12, 2019, https://www.peta.org/about-peta/faq/whats-wrong-with -wearing-wool/.

**49** "Highly Processed Foods Linked to Addictive Eating," University of Michigan (press release), February 18, 2015, https://news.umich .edu/highly-processed-foods-linked-to-addictive-eating/.

**50** Mueen Aslam and Walter Hurley, "Biological Activities of Peptides Derived from Milk Proteins," Illinois Livestock Trail, August 5, 1998, http://livestocktrail.illinois.edu/dairynet/paperDisplay.cfm?ContentI D=249.

**51** Neal Barnard, *Breaking the Food Seduction* (New York: St. Martin's Press, 2003), 63.

52 James Ponder, "Vegans Found to Have Highest Amount of Disease-Fighting Biomarkers," Loma Linda University Health, March 27, 2019, https://news.llu.edu/research/vegans-found-have-highest-amount-of-disease-fighting-biomarkers.

53 Nicholas Bakalar, "Getting Your Protein from Plants May Help You Live Longer," *New York Times*, updated September 9, 2019, https://www.nytimes.com/2019/09/03/well/eat/diet-lifespan-vegetables-vegetarian-vegan-foods-plants-meat-fish.html.

54 "Foods That Can Cause Food Poisoning," The Centers for Disease Control and Prevention, accessed November 2, 2019, https://www.cdc.gov/foodsafety/foods-linked-illness.html.

55 "Steroid Hormone Implants Used for Growth in Food-Producing Animals," U.S. Food & Drug Administration, accessed November 5, 2019, https://www.fda.gov/animal-veterinary/product-safety-information/steroid-hormone-implants-used-growth-food-producing-animals.

56 Daniel Patrick, "How Much Protein Do You Need Every Day?" Harvard Medical School, June 18, 2015, https://www.health.harvard.edu/blog/how-much-protein-do-you-need-every-day-201506188096.

57 McKenna Princing, "Could Some Gut Bacteria Cause Colon Cancer?" *Right as Rain*, April 9, 2018, https://rightasrain.uwmedicine.org/well/health/could-some-gut-bacteria-cause-colon-cancer.

58 Aleksandra Tomova, et al., "The Effects of Vegetarian and Vegan Diets on Gut Microbiota," *Frontiers in Nutrition* 6 (April 2019): 47.

59 Kate Good, "U.S. Factory Farms Produce Enough Waste to Fill the Empire State Building... Every Single Day!" One Green Planet, accessed October 5, 2019, https://www.onegreenplanet.org/news/u-s-factory-farm-waste/.

60 Maria Mirabelli, "Asthma Symptoms Among Adolescents Who Attend Public Schools That Are Located Near Confined Swine Feeding Operations," *Pediatrics* 118, no. 1 (July 2006): e66–e75.

61 Lauren Bonatakis, "Proper Land Management Can Offset Greenhouse Gas Emissions from Grass-Fed Cattle," Envirobites, August 28, 2019, https://envirobites.org/2019/08/28/proper-land-management-can-offset-greenhouse-gas-emissions-from-grass-fed-cattle/.

62 "Slaughterhouse Workers," Food Empowerment Project, accessed November 4, 2019, https://foodispower.org/human-labor-slavery/slaughterhouse-workers/.

63 Kathy Freston, "Vegan: Great for Kids!" *HuffPost*, October 5, 2011, https://www.huffpost.com/entry/vegan-kids-diet_b_877680.

**64** Michael Greger, "Heart Disease Starts in Childhood," NutritionFacts.org, September 23, 2013, https://nutritionfacts.org/video/heart-disease-starts-in-childhood/.

**65** European Society of Cardiology, "Low Carbohydrate Diets Are Unsafe and Should Be Avoided, Study Suggests," *ScienceDaily*, August 28, 2018, www.sciencedaily.com/releases/2018/08/180828085922.htm.

**66** Yvette Brazier, "How Safe is the Paleo Diet?" *Medical News Today*, February 19, 2016, https://www.medicalnewstoday.com/articles/306816.php.

**67** "Paleo Diet Increases Risk for Heart Disease," Physicians Committee for Responsible Medicine, July 25, 2019, https://www.pcrm.org/news/health-nutrition/paleo-diet-increases-risk-heart-disease.

**68** Scott Douglas, "How Paleo Diet Affects Lipid Levels," *Runner's World*, May 16, 2013, https://www.runnersworld.com/nutrition-weight-loss/a20797427/how-paleo-diet-affects-lipid-levels/.

**69** Margaret Murphy, et al., "Whole Beetroot Consumption Acutely Improves Running Performance," *Journal of the Academy of Nutrition and Dietetics* 112, no. 4 (April 2012): 548–52.

**70** Joel Eggebeen, et al., "One Week of Daily Dosing with Beetroot Juice Improves Submaximal Endurance and Blood Pressure in Older Patients with Heart Failure and Preserved Ejection Fraction," *JACC: Heart Failure* 4, no. 6 (February 2016): 428–37.

**71** "World Record Yoke Walk at Veg Fest by Vegan Patrik," Great Vegan Athletes, accessed July 29, 2019, https://www.greatveganathletes.com/news_articles/world-record-yoke-walk-at-veg-fest-by-vegan-patrik/.

**72** Marc Bekoff, "Pigs Are Intelligent, Emotional, and Cognitively Complex," *Psychology Today*, June 12, 2015, https://www.psychologytoday.com/us/blog/animal-emotions/201506/pigs-are-intelligent-emotional-and-cognitively-complex.

**73** Joanne Edgar, et al., "Avian Maternal Response to Chick Distress," *Proceedings of the Royal Society B* 278, no. 1721 (February 2011): 3129–134.

**74** Springer, "Think Chicken: Think Intelligent, Caring and Complex: Review Looks at Studies on Chicken Intelligence, Social Development and Emotions," *ScienceDaily*, August 28, 2018, www.sciencedaily.com/releases/2017/01/170103091955.html.

**75** Grant Gerlock, "Farmers Take Out Millions in Loans to Raise Chickens for Big-Box Retailers," *The Salt*, NPR, June 22, 2017, https://www.npr.org/sections/thesalt/2017/06/22/533944458/farmers-take-out-millions-in-loans-to-raise-chickens-for-big-box-retailers.

**76** "Cows Reacting to Live Music Performance Will Leave You In Awe," Rumble Viral, video, 2:47, April 12, 2016, https://www.youtube.com /watch?v=MFu2qN51zgg.

**77** Rhys Harrison, et al., "Blindness Caused by a Junk Food Diet," *Annals of Internal Medicine* 171, no. 11 (December 2019): 859–61.

**78** Australian Associated Press, "Vitamins and Antioxidants: Some Supplements Linked to Increased Risk of Death," *The Guardian*, May 28, 2018, https://www.theguardian.com/australia-news/2018 /may/29/vitamins-and-antioxidants-some-supplements-linked-to -increased-risk-of-death.

**79** Heike Bischoff-Ferrari, et al., "Calcium Intake and Hip Fracture Risk in Men and Women: A Meta-Analysis of Prospective Cohort Studies and Randomized Controlled Trials," *American Journal of Clinical Nutrition* 86, no. 6 (December 2007): 1780–790.

**80** Mark Hay, "This Is What Fish Oil Supplements Actually Do," *Vice*, May 17, 2019, https://www.vice.com/en_us/article/43jnyp/this-is -what-fish-oil-supplements-actually-do.

**81** Lauren Steussy, "Is Fish Oil the New Snake Oil? New Studies Debunk Omega-3 Hype," *New York Post*, August 30, 2019, https://nypost.com/2019/08/30/is-fish-oil-the-new-snake-oil-new -studies-debunk-the-omega-3-hype/.

**82** Michael Greger, "Vitamin B$_{12}$," NutritionFacts.org, accessed August 30, 2019, https://nutritionfacts.org/topics/vitamin-b12/.

**83** World Cancer Research Fund/American Institute for Cancer Research, "Food, Nutrition, Physical Activity, and the Prevention of Cancer: A Global Perspective," Washington, DC: AICR, 2007, http://discovery.ucl.ac.uk/4841/1/4841.pdf.

**84** Donna Winham and Andrea Hutchins, "Perceptions of Flatulence from Bean Consumption Among Adults in 3 Feeding Studies," *Nutrition Journal* 10 (November 2011): 128.

**85** Michael Rafii, "The Incalculable Cost of Alzheimer's," Alzheimer's Association, May 20, 2010, https://www.alz.org/blog/alz/may _2010/the_incalculable_cost_of_alzheimer_s.

**86** Northwestern University, "Higher Egg and Cholesterol Consumption Hikes Heart Disease and Early Death Risk," *ScienceDaily*, March 15, 2019, https://www.sciencedaily.com/releases/2019/03/1903151 10858.htm.

**87** "Lowering Cholesterol with a Plant-Based Diet," Physicians Committee for Responsible Medicine, accessed October 12, 2019, https://www.pcrm.org/good-nutrition/nutrition-information/lowering -cholesterol-with-a-plant-based-diet.

**88** "The Truth About Fats: The Good, the Bad, and the In-Between," Harvard Medical School, updated December 11, 2019, https://www.health.harvard.edu/staying-healthy/the-truth-about-fats-bad-and-good.

**89** Institute of Medicine, *Dietary Reference Intakes for Energy, Carbohydrate, Fiber, Fat, Fatty Acids, Cholesterol, Protein, and Amino Acids* (Washington, DC: The National Academies Press, 2005), https://www.nap.edu/catalog/10490/dietary-reference-intakes-for-energy-carbohydrate-fiber-fat-fatty-acids-cholesterol-protein-and-amino-acids.

**90** Ida Laake, et al., "A Prospective Study of Intake of Trans-Fatty Acids From Ruminant Fat, Partially Hydrogenated Vegetable Oils, and Marine Oils and Mortality from CVD," *British Nutrition Journal* 108, no. 4 (August 2012): 743–54.

**91** "Worldwide Toll of Diabetes," International Diabetes Federation, accessed May 20, 2020, https://diabetesatlas.org/en/sections/worldwide-toll-of-diabetes.html.

**92** "Statistics about Diabetes," American Diabetes Association, accessed October 2, 2019, https://www.diabetes.org/resources/statistics/statistics-about-diabetes.

**93** Christy Brissette, "Trying to Conceive? Think About What You're Eating," *Chicago Tribune*, July 27, 2017, https://www.chicagotribune.com/lifestyles/health/ct-nutrition-and-fertility-20170727-story.html.

**94** Jolynn Tumolo, "Saffron as Effective as Some Antidepressants," Psychiatry & Behavioral Health Learning Network, October 17, 2014, https://www.psychcongress.com/article/saffron-effective-some-antidepressants.

**95** Elizabeth Spencer, et al., "Diet and Body Mass Index in 38000 EPIC-Oxford Meat-Eaters, Fish-Eaters, Vegetarians and Vegans," *International Journal of Obesity and Related Metabolic Disorders* 27, no. 6 (June 2003): 728–34.

**96** Kate Volkman Oakes, "Can Wellness Cure?" University of California, San Francisco, May 30, 2013, https://www.ucsf.edu/news/2013/05/105701/can-wellness-cure.

**97** Dean Ornish, et al., "Effect of Comprehensive Lifestyle Changes on Telomerase Activity and Telomere Length in Men with Biopsy-Proven Low-Risk Prostate Cancer: 5-year Follow-Up of a Descriptive Pilot Study," *The Lancet Oncology* 14, no. 11 (October 2013): 1112–120.

**98** Becky Little, "When Cigarette Companies Used Doctors to Push Smoking," HISTORY, updated September 11, 2019, https://www.history.com/news/cigarette-ads-doctors-smoking-endorsement.

**99** Sara Miller, "There Are Nearly 1 Billion Smokers on Earth," *Live Science*, April 5, 2017, https://www.livescience.com/58563 -one-billion-smokers.html.

**100** Alastair Bland, "Is the Livestock Industry Destroying the Planet?" *Smithsonian Magazine*, August 1, 2012, https://www.smithsonianmag .com/travel/is-the-livestock-industry-destroying-the-planet-11308007/.

**101** Jeff Stein, "Congress Just Passed an $867 Billion Farm Bill. Here's What's In It," *Washington Post*, December 12, 2019, https://www.washingtonpost.com/business/2018/12/11 /congresss-billion-farm-bill-is-out-heres-whats-it/.

**102** David Simon, *Meatonomics: How the Rigged Economics of Meat and Dairy Make You Consume Too Much* (San Francisco: Conari Press, 2013), 80.

**103** "Crop Acreage Data," USDA Farm Service Agency, accessed July 22, 2019, http://www.fsa.usda.gov/FSA/webapp?area=newsro om&subject=landing&topic=foi-er-fri-cad.

**104** Simon, *Meatonomics*, xv.

**105** Samantha Raphelson, "Nobody Is Moving Our Cheese: American Surplus Reaches Record High," *Here & Now*, NPR, January 9, 2019, https://www.npr.org/2019/01/09/683339929 /nobody-is-moving-our-cheese-american-surplus-reaches-record-high.

**106** Arthur Allen, "U.S. Touts Fruit and Vegetables While Subsidizing Animals That Become Meat," *Washington Post,* October 3, 2011, https://www.washingtonpost.com/national/health-science/us-touts -fruit-and-vegetables-while-subsidizing-animals-that-become-meat /2011/08/22/gIQATFG5IL_story.html.

**107** Bo Ra Lee, et al., "Effects of 12-Week Vegetarian Diet on the Nutritional Status, Stress Status and Bowel Habits in Middle School Students and Teachers," *Clinical Nutritional Research* 5, no. 2 (April 2016): 102–11.

**108** Jennifer Hyland, "Fast Fiber Facts: What It Is and How to Get Enough," *US News and World Report*, August 22, 2018, https://health.usnews.com/health-care/for-better/articles/2018-08 -22/fast-fiber-facts-what-it-is-and-how-to-get-enough.

**109** Sally Wadyka, "A Healthier Way to Get More Protein," Consumer Reports, August 2, 2019, https://www.consumerreports .org/nutrition-healthy-eating/healthier-way-to-get-more-protein-plant -sources/.

**110** "Laxatives OTC Revenue in the United States from 2015 to 2018," *Statista*, accessed May 18, 2020, https://www.statista.com /statistics/506583/otc-revenue-of-laxatives-in-the-us/.

**111** Melanie Joy, *Why We Love Dogs, Eat Pigs, and Wear Cows: An Introduction to Carnism* (San Francisco: Red Wheel, 2011), 27–28.

**112** "California Wildlife Win Protections from Federal Trapping, Gunning," Center for Biological Diversity (press release), November 1, 2017, https://www.biologicaldiversity.org/news/press_releases /2017/wildlife-services-11-01-2017.php.

**113** "Cruel Wildlife Trapping," PETA, accessed September 5, 2019, https://www.peta.org/issues/wildlife/cruel-wildlife-control/cruel -wildlife-trapping/.

**114** "Researchers Say Most Alzheimer's Disease Cases Are Preventable—Find Out How," Blue Zones, accessed October 2, 2019, https://www.bluezones.com/2017/09/researchers-say-alzheimers -disease-cases-preventable-find/.

**115** Lindsay Oberst, "New Book Shows How 90% of Alzheimer's Cases Are Preventable," Food Revolution Network, September 13, 2017, https://foodrevolution.org/blog/food-and-health/prevent -reverse-alzheimers/.

**116** LJ Gambone, "Loma Linda Doctors Say You Can Prevent or Turn Around Alzheimer's Disease," *Daily Press*, updated May 15, 2018, https://www.vvdailypress.com/news/20180509/loma-linda-doctors -say-you-can-prevent-or-turn-around-alzheimers-disease.

**117** Jihad Alwarith, et al., "Nutrition Interventions in Rheumatoid Arthritis: The Potential Use of Plant-Based Diets. A Review," *Frontiers in Nutrition* 6 (September 2019): 141.

**118** Chelsea Clinton, et al., "Whole-Foods, Plant-Based Diet Alleviates the Symptoms of Osteoarthritis," *Hindawi*, February 28, 2015, https://www.arthritis.org/health-wellness/healthy-living/nutrition /anti-inflammatory/vegetarian-diet-arthritis.

**119** "High-Fiber Diet Lowers Risk for Arthritis," Physicians Committee for Responsible Medicine, May 24, 2017, https://www.pcrm.org /news/health-nutrition/high-fiber-diet-lowers-risk-arthritis.

**120** "Arthritis: Reduce Arthritis Pain with a Plant-Based Diet," Physicians Committee for Responsible Medicine, accessed August 5, 2019, https://www.pcrm.org/health-topics/arthritis.

**121** Carl Safina, "Are We Wrong to Assume Fish Can't Feel Pain?" *Guardian*, October 30, 2018, https://www.theguardian.com/news /2018/oct/30/are-we-wrong-to-assume-fish-cant-feel-pain.

**122** "Fish: A Silent Scream," International Organization for Animal Protection, June 17, 2016, https://www.oipa.org/international/fish -a-silent-scream/.

**123** Jonathan Balcombe, "Do Fish Feel Pain?" *Nature* (blog), PBS, July 19, 2017, http://www.pbs.org/wnet/nature/blog/fish-feel-pain/.

# About the Authors

**GENE STONE** (GeneStone.com) is a former Peace Corps volunteer, journalist, and book, magazine, and newspaper editor, as well as a *New York Times* bestselling author. He has written, cowritten, or ghostwritten more than forty-five books on a wide variety of subjects, but for the last decade he has concentrated on plant-based diets and their relationship to health, animal protection, and the environment. Among these books are *Forks Over Knives*, *How Not to Die*, *Animalkind*, *The Awareness*, *The Engine 2 Diet*, *Living the Farm Sanctuary Life*, *Rescue Dogs*, *Mercy for Animals*, *Healthy at Last*, and *Eat for the Planet*.

**KATHY FRESTON** (KathyFreston.com) is a *New York Times* bestselling author of multiple health and wellness books, notably *The Lean*, *Quantum Wellness*, and *Clean Protein*. Her advocacy for a more healthy, sustainable, and just food system is inspired by her concern for human health as well as animal and environmental welfare. Kathy appears frequently on national TV, including *Ellen*, *The Dr. Oz Show*, *Good Morning America*, *The Talk*, *Extra*, and *Oprah*, and her work has been featured in *Vanity Fair*, *Harper's Bazaar*, *Self*, *W*, *Fitness*, and *HuffPost*. Kathy enjoys hiking and biking, will travel almost anywhere for a good vegan meal, and is obsessed with her adopted dog, Trixie.